COVID- 19 VIRUS, WHAT IS THE PERPETUAL WAY OUT?

I0758956

FIND THE ASTONISHING MYSTERIES TO BOOSTING YOUR IMMUNITY AND CARRYING ON WITH A INFECTIONS FREE LIFE, PRESENTLY AND LATER ON

TOM DAVIES

COPYRIGHT©2021

ALL RIGHT RESERVED

TABLE OF CONTENTS

INTRODUCTION

CHAPTER ONE

WATER

CHAPTER TWO

ZINC AND MAGNESIUM
INSTANCES OF FOOD VARIETIES AND NATURAL PRODUCTS WEALTHY IN ZINC
MEDICAL AND NUTRITIONAL BENEFITS
MAGNESIUM AND YOUR WELLBEING
FOOD SOURCES AND ORGANIC PRODUCTS WEALTHY IN MAGNESIUM

CHAPTER THREE

RESISTANT BOOSTING FOOD SOURCES AND NATURAL PRODUCTS
VITAMIN D RICH FOOD SOURCES
SOURCES OF VITAMIN D
VITAMIN D FOOD VARIETIES

CHAPTER FOUR

IMMUNE BOOSTING FOOD VARIETIES AND ORGANIC PRODUCTS
VITAMIN C AND E RICH FOOD VARIETIES
LEAFY FOODS THAT HAVE MORE VITAMIN C THAN ORANGE
FOOD SOURCES AND NATURAL PRODUCTS RICH IN VITAMIN E

INTRODUCTION

The world was quite somewhat as far as bacterial and viral control and its residents were approaching their different undertakings and sometimes interests until a tempest struck it.

It happens in mid-November 2019 at a fish market in a country area called Wuhan in the Hubei Province in China.

Although China specifically and the world, when all is said in done, attempted to make light of the seriousness of the infection, it blew in our appearances before we knew it

This book will zero in on the utilization of nourishment through plant-based and animal-based food varieties for upgrading immunity as well as to construct a solid safeguard for all class of individuals from the matured to the more youthful individual against COVID-19 as well as against all kind of sickness and infections both in the short and in the long run. In people, Covid-19 is remembered for the range of infections that cause the regular cold and as of late, serious intense respiratory disorder (SARS). Arising irresistible illnesses, for example, SARS presents a significant danger to general wellbeing. The tale of Covid-19 has spread quickly to numerous nations and has been proclaimed a pandemic by the World Health Organization. COVID-19 is generally brought about by an infection to which most presumably individuals with low resistance reaction are being influenced. Plant-based food varieties increased the intestinal advantageous microscopic organisms which are useful and comprise 85% of the immunity framework. By the utilization of a lot of water, minerals like magnesium and Zinc, micronutrients, spices, food rich in vitamin C, D, and E, and a superior way of life, one can advance wellbeing and can conquer this disease. Different examinations explored that an amazing cell reinforcement glutathione and bioflavonoid quercetin may forestall different contaminations including COVID-19. Taking everything into account, plant-based food sources assume an indispensable part to upgrade the immunity of individuals to control COVID-19.

Covid-19 assaults individuals with low safe frameworks and individuals particularly individuals of underage and overages. The safe framework is based on the useful live bacterium that lives in the gut which shields the human body from different infections. At the point when the safe framework reaction is low, feeble, or harmed, it turns into an open greeting for contaminations, for example, Covid-19 or different infections like diabetes, coronary illness, or malignancy. Plant-based food varieties increase and help the intestinal gainful microscopic organisms and the general gut micro biome wellbeing which makes up to 85% of the body's immunity framework. Then again, an overabundance of animal-based food sources drains the group of good microbes, advances aggravation, which is the basic reason for diabetes, persistent obstructive aspiratory illness cardiovascular infections, hepatitis B, malignancy, and constant kidney sicknesses.

CHAPTER ONE

WATER

*P*atients of Covid-19 should have a lot of water, as that will keep their mucous layers clammy which can additionally bring down the odds of cold and influenza. Assuming they do not detect thirst that much, they can plan soup for them or have coconut water, milk, green tea, and surprisingly some custom-made organic product juice will be useful. There is right now no proof of the infection endurance in sewage or drinking water.

The COVID-19 infection's morphological qualities and compound synthesis are like any other human proxy infection on which information is accessible to both manageability in the climate and proficient coagulation measure.

A fantasy that consumable water should keep Covid-19 under control like clockwork had been running in the features around the planet a couple of days prior. Although drinking water does not guarantee that you would not be infected with the virus, staying hydrated can improve your wellbeing and ensure the insusceptible framework can overcome the infection if it is moved to you. Drinking water attempts to assist your cells with oxygenating. Cells can contend at their best if they get sufficient oxygen that assists them with shielding the body from any irresistible specialists that endeavor to enter, or on the off chance that they do, they battle them.

As indicated by clinical specialists, hydration frequently assumes a significant part in checking your internal heat level. Be that as it may, if you have a fever, if it is a result of COVID-19 or some other contamination or turmoil in the body, drinking a lot of water is truly significant. Drinking sufficient water is fundamental, for a lot of reasons, as demonstrated in a Clinical Wellbeing report, keeping the danger of illness brought down is one of them. Remaining hydrated likewise empowers the transmission of supplements to all pieces of the body and assists with keeping up all body capacities and organs working possibly to diminish body contamination. Dryness in the bodies can be brought about by the medications we take on the off chance that we have infection contamination—like basic cold, and influenza. At the point when we are wiped out, we begin losing a large part of the body's water as a bodily fluid, and that is how our body eliminates the infection-causing microbes from the body. Until we drink a lot of water, we stay hydrated, and we can eliminate more bodily fluid (alongside germs) from our bodies.

Until we get a fix and a more viable novel Covid-19 immunization other than the oxford Astra-Zeneca antibodies and it likes that is being encircled by discussions over its viability and likely notions from across the world, taking every single preventive measure and protecting ourselves is pivotal. Although drinking bunches of water does not promise that you would not be infected with the novel virus, it very well may be powerful in diminishing your peril generally, and can likewise assist you with recuperating after the sickness.

CHAPTER TWO

ZINC AND MAGNESIUM

A fundamental micronutrient is utilized in DNA amalgamation and cell expansion. It is additionally engaged with the guideline of intrinsic and versatile resistant reactions, cell flagging, and the creation of insusceptible cells. Food varieties that contain Zinc incorporate red meat and shellfish.

An extremely essential mineral for our insusceptible framework, magnesium, is likewise a significant electrolyte that assists our body with reinforcing our safe framework's characteristic executioner cells and lymphocytes. It is likewise a vital wellspring of energy for our bodies called adenosine triphosphate (ATP), which is significant to the point that without this energy, our body cannot work as expected. Magnesium helps the hemoglobin in our blood which is answerable for conveying oxygen from our lungs to the whole human body which aids COVID-19 contamination since the infection assaults the respiratory framework. Food varieties wealthy in magnesium are dull chocolate, dark beans, avocados, and entire grains.

INSTANCES OF FOOD VARIETIES AND NATURAL PRODUCTS WEALTHY IN ZINC

Animal food sources are the best wellsprings of zinc compared to plant food sources, similar to vegetables since zinc bioavailability (the small part of zinc that is held and utilized by the body) is high in food sources like meat and fish.

This is because of the shortfall of mixtures that repress zinc ingestion in animal food sources and the presence of sulfur-containing amino acids that improve zinc assimilation, similar to cysteine and methionine.

Although there are plant-based zinc food sources, they're less bio-accessible as a result of their high substance of phytic corrosive (or phytates), which hinders zinc assimilation.

Reports propose that individuals who do not eat meat or related items, similar to individuals on a veggie lover or vegetarian diet, need up to 50 percent more zinc in their eating regimens to assimilate what the body needs.

Be that as it may, the inhibitory impacts of phytic corrosive on the retention of zinc can be limited with strategies like drenching, warming, growing, aging, and raising. Research additionally shows that the assimilation of zinc can be improved by utilizing yeast-based bread and sourdough bread, sprouts, and presoaked vegetables.

The most ideal approach to accomplish ideal zinc levels is to burn-through a few servings of these zinc food sources each day:

1. SHEEP

Sheep is a rich wellspring of numerous nutrients minerals. Notwithstanding zinc, sheep contains nutrient B12, riboflavin, selenium, niacin, phosphorus, and iron.

2. PUMPKIN SEEDS

Pumpkin seeds and pumpkin seed oil are demonstrated to be vital nourishment for keeping up wellbeing in post-menopausal ladies. Pumpkin seeds are additionally useful for prostate wellbeing, and they advance your psychological well-being.

3. HEMP SEEDS

Not exclusively are hemp seeds wealthy in zinc, yet they are an incredible wellspring of omega-3 and omega-6 unsaturated fats, which effects affect your cardiovascular framework and assists with keeping aggravation under control.

4. GRASS-FED BEEF

Grass-fed beef sustenance incorporates omega-3 unsaturated fats and formed linoleic corrosive, an amazing polyunsaturated unsaturated fat that has been appeared to help decrease the danger of coronary illness, improve glucose, debilitate weight gain, and construct muscle.

5. CHICKPEAS (GARBANZO BEANS)

Chickpeas, similar to all vegetables, are a type of complex sugars that the body can gradually process and use for energy. Studies show that chickpeas increase satiety and help with weight reduction. They additionally improve assimilation by rapidly moving food sources through the stomach-related lot.

6. LENTILS

Lentils are known for their well-being advancing impacts, as they are rich in polyphenols and micronutrients, including zinc. Lentils fill in as a plant-based protein, making them phenomenal zinc-rich nourishment for veggie lovers.

7. COCOA POWDER

Cocoa powder is a decent wellspring of two flavonoids, epicatechin, and catechin, which work as cell reinforcements that help forestall aggravation and infection. Due to the presence of flavonoids in cocoa powder, it improves the bloodstream and lowers pulse as well.

8. CASHEWS

Cashews are wealthy in unsaturated fats and high in protein. Cashews sustenance helps battle coronary illness, decrease irritation, advance bone wellbeing, and backing sound mind work. These nuts assist with weight reduction or support since they cause you to feel fuller and control food longings. Cashews have great zinc to copper proportion, to help guarantee that both of these minerals stay in balance.

9. KEFIR OR YOGURT

Kefir and yogurt are refined dairy items that fill in as probiotic food varieties. Both kefir and probiotic yogurt support solid assimilation, help the resistant framework, advance cardiovascular wellbeing, and direct your disposition.

10. RICOTTA CHEDDAR

Ricotta cheddar is one of the best cheddar choices since it contains striking measures of sound unsaturated fats and micronutrients, including zinc. Contrasted with numerous different sorts of cheddar, ricotta is likewise lower in sodium and soaked fat, and it's viewed as a "new cheddar" since it's not matured.

11. MUSHROOMS

Demonstrated mushroom sustenance benefits incorporate the capacity to support insusceptibility because of its cancer prevention agent exercises and diminish irritation.

12. SPINACH

Spinach is quite possibly the most supplement-thick food source in the present. It contains extraordinary defensive carotenoids that have been connected with diminishing the danger of numerous infections, including coronary illness, stoutness, diabetes, neurodegenerative sicknesses, and surprisingly more.

13. AVOCADO

In case you're searching for natural products that contain zinc, go after an avocado. It's known as probably the best food on earth since it's loaded with fundamental supplements. Also, research shows that avocado utilization is related to better eating routine quality and supplement consumption.

14. CHICKEN

Notwithstanding the zinc present in chicken, it's likewise a decent wellspring of B nutrients, including vitamin B12, niacin, nutrient B6, and pantothenic corrosive. The vitamin B12 in chicken keeps up energy levels, supports disposition, keeps up heart wellbeing, and lift skin wellbeing.

15. ALMONDS

Pondering which nuts are high in zinc? Almonds sustenance is really wonderful and numerous examinations show that it benefits numerous parts of wellbeing including cardiovascular wellbeing and weight control. Notwithstanding their zinc content, almonds likewise give nutrients E, manganese, magnesium, and riboflavin, among other significant micronutrients.

16. OATS

Could you ask for anything better about cereal? It's reasonable, flexible, and interminably comfortable. In addition to the fact that oats contain solvent fiber, which has been connected to a brought down hazard of coronary illness yet a large portion of a cup likewise contains 1.3 milligrams of zinc which is 16% of a lady's day by day need. Consider it one more motivation to cherish the exemplary breakfast staple.

17. SHELLFISH

Per ounce, shellfish have the most elevated zinc convergence of any food. Three ounces of crude clams contain 32 milligrams of zinc; multiple occasions the suggested day-by-day admission for the normal lady.

Another advantage: That equivalent measure of clams likewise contains more than 100% of your day-by-day needs for vitamin B12, which is significant for your sensory system, digestion, and sound platelets.

18. LEAN MEAT

Although specialists prescribe restricting red meat utilization to close to a couple of times each week, a lean hamburger can in any case be a solid piece of your eating regimen.

Select 95% lean ground meat or lean cuts (like sirloin) with the fat managed and you'll score 5.7 milligrams of zinc per four-ounce serving. That is a little more than 70% of the suggested everyday esteem.

19. CRAB

Pounding the meat out of entire bubbled crabs or do you favor the straightforwardness and delightful flavoring of singed crab cakes?

In any case, three ounces of cooked crab meat contains up to 7 milligrams of zinc, around 88% of what ladies need in a day. While the specific measure of zinc you'll get changes from one animal category to another, all crabs are extraordinary wellsprings of the mineral.

20. DARK BEANS

Another magnificent plant-based wellspring of zinc, Dark beans. Prepare a cup of cooked dark beans on top of that serving of mixed greens and you'll get 2 milligrams of zinc or 25% of your everyday needs. These beans are additionally high in iron, phosphorus, calcium, and magnesium, which support generally speaking wellbeing and are particularly significant for bone wellbeing.

21. GREEK YOGURTS

Greek yogurt has so numerous heavenly medical advantages and here one more one to add to the rundown: a seven-ounce compartment of plain, low-fat Greek yogurt packs 1.5 milligrams of zinc which is 19% of what a lady needs every day. It's likewise wealthy in absorption boosting probiotics.

22. SESAME SEEDS

Sesame seeds are additionally an incredible wellspring of phytosterols, intensifies that help lower cholesterol. Another compound in sesame seeds, called sesamin, helps balance chemicals and lifts general wellbeing. The seeds are likewise high in protein You can utilize sesame seed margarine in the spot of peanut butter on your toast. The seeds additionally pair very well with salmon or chicken – you can make heavenly custom-made granola.

23. FLAX SEEDS

Flax seeds are additionally amazingly wealthy in omega-3 unsaturated fats – supplements that support heart and cerebrum wellbeing – as well as offering various advantages. The seeds additionally help in the treatment of joint pain and incendiary inside infection

You can add ground flax seeds to your morning meal smoothies or plates of mixed greens. You can likewise sprinkle the seeds on cooked vegetables.

24. SWISS CHEDDAR

Note that cheddar is one solid wellspring of calcium – the mineral you need for solid bones. What's more, since it is a creature source, Swiss cheddar is viewed as a total protein – it contains every one of the amino acids your body needs to make protein.

In any case, practice control as Swiss cheddar additionally contains soaked fat that may not be sound whenever taken in huge sums.

You can add a cut of Swiss cheddar to your sandwich or bowl of soup. Add destroyed cheddar to your vegetable serving of mixed greens. Or then again have it with fried eggs.

25. EGG YOLK

Egg yolk is packed with different supplements also. It contains nutrients A, D, E, and K. The yolk is additionally wealthy in omega-3 unsaturated fats. Also, more significantly, the yolk contains the cancer prevention agents lutein and zeaxanthin – intensifies that support vision wellbeing

Bubbled egg yolk is a decent alternative – you can add it to your serving of mixed greens.

26. LIMA BEANS

Aside from zinc, lima beans are additionally wealthy in folate – a supplement needed for DNA union and cell division The beans are likewise plentiful in nutrients B1 and B6 and the fiber in the beans ensures the colon and battles stomach related diseases. It additionally can advance satiety and in the long run, energize solid weight reduction.

You can add dried lima beans to your evening bowl of soup. A blend of bacon and eggs with lima beans simply sounds so awesome.

27. KIDNEY BEANS

Aside from assisting you with getting sufficient measures of zinc, kidney beans likewise lessen the centralizations of C-receptive protein which is known to cause provocative problems. The beans likewise control glucose levels and perpetually help in the treatment of diabetes.

They can be a straightforward expansion to your ordinary natural product or vegetable serving of mixed greens. Or on the other hand, you can have canned beans as a sound evening nibble. In any event, adding them to good soups or stews can function admirably.

28. PEANUTS

Peanuts are additionally a host to a few heart-sound supplements. These incorporate niacin, magnesium, copper, oleic corrosive and different cancer prevention agents incorporate all-famous resveratrol.

Nut utilization has additionally been connected to a diminished danger of gallstone improvement in the two people. This could be ascribed to the cholesterol-bringing down impacts of peanuts as gallstones are for the most part made of cholesterol.

Eating them directly out of the shell could be the most ideal way. Breaking and nibbling, as we can likewise call it. Get a modest bunch of peanuts as you sit to watch the evening sitcom – and indeed, break and bite.

Or then again pause; you can likewise add peanuts to granola bar plans.

29. GARLIC

The best advantage garlic has is for the heart. This (alongside its different advantages) can be credited to allicin, a compound that displays intense natural impacts. Furthermore, regardless of being exceptionally nutritious, garlic has many calories. It can improve circulatory strain and cholesterol levels. It can battle the normal virus. Its cell reinforcements additionally help forestall psychological decay all the more strangely; garlic can likewise help detoxify the weighty metals inside the body.

Garlic is best burned-through crude – when you strip the cloves and eat them. This could be hard for the vast majority, given its impactful flavor. You can likewise smash the garlic and blend it in with nectar and spread on your toast – and chomp your approach to wonderful wellbeing.

30. BROWN COLORED RICE (COOKED)

Earthy-colored rice is additionally wealthy in manganese, which helps supplement assimilation and the creation of stomach-related proteins. Manganese additionally fortifies the resistant framework.

Earthy-colored rice is likewise known to control glucose levels and help in diabetes treatment.

You can supplant white rice with earthy colored rice in your dishes.

31. TURKEY

Turkey is wealthy in protein, which can build satiety and keep you full for significant stretches. This can debilitate indulging. Getting sufficient protein can likewise keep insulin levels stable after suppers.

Furthermore, actually like chicken, the selenium in turkey may help decline the danger of various sorts of disease

It's in every case best to go for a new, lean, field-raised turkey that is low in sodium. Eating the entire turkey can be a decent and belly-filling bargain.

32. MUSHROOMS

Mushrooms are probably the most uncommon wellspring of germanium, a supplement that assists your body with using oxygen adequately. Mushrooms likewise give iron and nutrients C and D.

Adding mushrooms to your soup can take it to an unheard-of level. You can prepare a couple of mushrooms for your vegetable serving of mixed greens. Or then again even add them to your curry.

MEDICAL AND NUTRITIONAL BENEFITS

1. Devouring food sources of zinc consistently will assist with improving your wellbeing in the accompanying manners.

2. WORKS AS AMAZING CELL REINFORCEMENT

Zinc assists with battling oxidative pressure and diminishes your odds of building up a few genuine infections. Research discovery founds that zinc supplementation essentially brought down contamination rates in members' ages 55 to 87 years.

3. BOOSTS EYE WELLBEING

Zinc is expected to change over Vitamin A into its dynamic structure to keep up legitimate vision. Sufficient admission of food varieties high in zinc can help improve night vision and the sky is the limit from there. This is because of zinc's capacity to lessen oxidation and aggravation, which are related to reduce eye wellbeing.

4• ENHANCES INSUSCEPTIBLE CAPACITY

The body needs zinc to initiate Lymphocytes, which are basic for legitimate invulnerable capacity and that is the reason individuals who are lacking in zinc keep an eye on more areas of defense to an assortment of ailments including the basic virus.

5• PROMOTES WOUND RECUPERATING

Zinc benefits the respectability of the skin and helps treat contaminations. Research shows that individuals who have deferred wound mending will in general have low degrees of zinc.

6• BALANCES CHEMICALS AND SUPPORTS REGENERATIVE WELLBEING

Zinc assumes a significant part in chemical creation. It's required for the creation of estrogen and progesterone in ladies, and it expands testosterone levels and sperm quality normally. Zinc is additionally expected to adjust insulin, the fundamental chemical associated with the guideline of ordinary glucose.

7• PROMOTES MUSCLE DEVELOPMENT

Zinc assumes a significant part in cell division and cell development, so it's expected to keep up the strength in the solid and skeletal frameworks. Zinc additionally assists with the arrival of testosterone, development chemical, and insulin-like development factor-1, all of which construct bulk and assist you with keeping sound digestion.

8• AIDS IN SUPPLEMENT RETENTION

Zinc influences protein union and is required by the body to utilize amino acids from food. It's likewise associated with the breakdown of sugars from food varieties, which are a portion of the fundamental wellsprings of energy from the body. This is the reason zinc inadequacy can prompt low energy levels and add to adrenal or ongoing weakness.

9• PROMOTES HEART WELLBEING

Zinc is expected to keep up the soundness of cells inside the cardiovascular framework, while likewise bringing down aggravation and oxidative pressure.

MAGNESIUM AND YOUR WELLBEING

Magnesium is a mineral that assumes a major part in making your body work right. Above 300 substance responses within you rely upon the mineral.

Without it, your muscles cannot move how they should. Your nerves would not send and get messages. Magnesium additionally keeps your heartbeat consistent, glucose levels adjusted, and your joint ligament solid. It helps your body make protein, bone and DNA.

Your body does not make magnesium all alone. The sum you need relies upon your age and sex. In case you're a lady age 19 or more established, you need 310 milligrams (mg) a day - 350 mg in case you're pregnant. In case you're a grown-up man under age 30, you need 400 mg daily. After 30, men need 420 mg.

It's in every case best to get magnesium from food; however, you can likewise get it from multivitamins and enhancements. To an extreme however can cause sickness, stomach issues, or runs. In outrageous cases, it could cause an unpredictable heartbeat or heart failure.

Try not to take a magnesium supplement if you have certain conditions, for example,

- Heart attack

- Kidney failure

- Bowel obstacle

- Myasthenia gravis

If you get a lot of magnesium from food, your kidneys will eliminate it through your urine. Your kidneys will likewise adjust your magnesium levels on the off chance that you do not get enough of it for a brief period.

Certain conditions like Crohn's illness, celiac infection, type 2 diabetes, liquor addiction, and persistent looseness of the bowels can give your body a drawn-out lack of magnesium. Regular indications incorporate loss of craving, sickness, spewing, and weariness

Verdant green vegetables, entire grains, beans, nuts, and fish are the most ideal approaches to keep sound degree of magnesium in your body. Shop in light of these points of interest:

FOOD SOURCES AND ORGANIC PRODUCTS WEALTHY IN MAGNESIUM

• Green verdant vegetables (for example spinach and kale)

• Fruit (figs, avocado, banana, and raspberries)

• Nuts and seeds

• Legumes (dark beans, chickpeas, and kidney beans)

• Vegetables (peas, broccoli, cabbage, green beans, artichokes, asparagus, Brussels sprouts)

- Seafood (salmon, mackerel, fish)

- Whole grains (earthy colored rice and oats)

- Raw cacao

- Dark Chocolate

- Tofu

- Baked beans

- Chlorella powder

FISH

Top Source of Magnesium

These sorts of fish are swimming in the mineral magnesium:

- Chinook salmon

- Halibut

- Atlantic mackerel

- Atlantic Pollock

Vegetables and Natural products wealthy in Magnesium

Thorny pear has a ton of magnesium, however, it is not the most effortless food to discover or get ready.

Zero in rather on these products of the soil that have a great deal of magnesium when you cook them and a lot of different supplements, as well:

- Spinach

- Swiss chard

- Edamame

- Tamarind

- Potato with skin

- Okra

ALGAE CAL

 Besides it is produced using Lithothamnion suppositum, a special strain of red sea green growth found on the shores of South America. What makes this green growth so uncommon is that it's unbelievably supplemented thick. Truth be told, it contains every one of the 13 fundamental bone-supporting minerals! Also, that incorporates a solid portion of magnesium.

This little sea plant is processed into a nutritious entire food powder. At that point, we add some additional magnesium to guarantee the ideal 2:1 proportion of calcium to magnesium is met. So a day-by-day portion of Algae Cal in addition to conveys 720 mg of calcium and 350 mg of magnesium including 11 other bone-supporting minerals and nutrients C, D, and K2!)

DARK CHOCOLATE

Dark chocolate is a definitive bliss food. Furthermore, not because it's flavorful! Chocolate really contains phenylethylamine, a characteristic chemical-like substance that causes the arrival of endorphins, your "vibe great" synapses.

Dark chocolate is additionally notable for its polyphenol cancer prevention agents that lower cholesterol and lift heart wellbeing. What's more, the cocoa in chocolate is very high in magnesium. For every 100 grams of dim chocolate (70-85% cocoa), there's around 228 mg of magnesium. That is more than 70% of your RDA. So appreciate it yet with some restraint obviously!

WHITE BEANS

White beans are an astounding wellspring of magnesium, fiber, and folate included. For every 100 grams of white beans (that is around ½ cup), you get an incredible 190 mg of magnesium.

Likewise, a high admission of beans is connected to essentially bring down dangers of coronary illness, hypertension, stroke, and type II diabetes. Note that different vegetables like naval force beans, pinto beans, and fava beans are likewise extraordinary wellsprings of magnesium.

DARK BEANS

Like different vegetables, dark beans are a veggie-lover staple since they're high in protein and low in fat and cholesterol. Besides, they're a rich wellspring of magnesium: 100grams contains 171 mg.

Dark beans help reinforce bones because their magnesium is joined with loads of calcium and phosphorus. They help oversee diabetes because their fiber improves glucose levels. What's more, they contain cancer prevention agents that are useful for your heart!

Take a stab at cooking them yourself by splashing them short-term. This lessens salt and builds flavor contrasted with canned beans.

PUMPKIN AND SQUASH SEEDS

Pumpkin and squash seeds are an amazingly nutritious tidbit. They're incredibly high in magnesium: 1 ounce (that is around 142 seeds) conveys 168 mg.

They additionally offer 30 grams of protein and 8 mg of iron. Furthermore, because these seeds have significant levels of amino corrosive tryptophan, eating a modest bunch around evening time can help you unwind.

PLANTAIN

Plantains are a staple for a huge number of individuals in tropical nations since they're a thick wellspring of boring energy. They're not difficult to plan as well. Basically cut them up, and sear them for a delectable tidbit!

Furthermore, only one plantain gives 109 mg of magnesium. These scrumptious natural products are likewise stacked with iron, potassium, and nutrient A, which all have bone medical advantages as well. Also, they're plentiful in B nutrients, especially B6, which can help lessen pressure side effects and cardiovascular infection hazards.

MACKEREL

As well as being an extraordinary wellspring of bone-solid omega 3 unsaturated fats, cold-water greasy fish like mackerel add more magnesium to your menu. Every 100 grams of mackerel (that is around one little filet), contains 97 mg of magnesium.

Mackerel is a significant wellspring of Vitamin B12, the difficult-to-get Vitamin B frequently connected with red meat. Try not to dismiss canned mackerel either — it offers a similar measure of minerals and nutrients as new fish. Simply know that canned fish regularly contains more sodium than new fish, so check your marks at the supermarket!

SPINACH

Spinach is loaded with magnesium, particularly when it's cooked. This is basically because cooked spinach withers down to a lot more modest size than crude spinach. For instance, a pound of crude spinach cooks down to only one cup, so you're getting the dietary substance of an entire pound of the vegetable yet burning-through a more modest sum! Furthermore, cooked spinach gives 87 mg of magnesium for every 100 grams, which is somewhat more than a large portion of a cup.

This green super food is likewise known for its high iron substance. You can improve your assimilation of iron from spinach by eating it close by vegetables plentiful in nutrient C (otherwise called ascorbic corrosive) like broccoli, Brussels fledglings, and cauliflower.

 Note: this idea applies to different vegetables wealthy in iron as well!

SWISS CHARD

You may have heard that dim, verdant greens are super food. That is because they're wealthy in supplements, similar to magnesium. What's more, Swiss chard is no special case. Every 100 grams (somewhat less than two cups) of cooked Swiss chard conveys an amazing 86 mg of magnesium. This vegetable is a brilliant wellspring of bone-solid nutrients A, K, and C!

ALMONDS

In case you're avoiding nuts since you're watching your weight, you'll be satisfied to realize almonds are among the least calorie nuts (164 calories for each ounce). They're likewise high in bone-building supplements like calcium and magnesium.

One ounce of almonds (a huge modest bunch) contains 76.5 mg of magnesium and 76.3 mg of calcium. Truth be told, almonds have more calcium and magnesium than some other nut! Almonds give protein and heart-sound fats. They additionally score high in Vitamin E and manganese — that equivalent modest bunch of almonds offers over 33% of the everyday prerequisites for every one of these supplements.

CASHEWS

Cashews are another nut wealthy in magnesium. For each one ounce of cashews (around 18 nuts), you get 73.7 mg of magnesium! Cashews might be high in carbs, yet they compensate for it by likewise being exceptionally nutritious. Notwithstanding magnesium, they're a decent wellspring of Vitamin E, K, and B-6, just as minerals like potassium and iron.

FIGS

You can eat figs dried or fresh; however, dried figs offer a wonderful surface and sweet flavor, in contrast to the fresh natural products. Furthermore, as well as being a scrumptious bite, figs have a ton to bring to the table regarding sustenance.

In particular, figs are a decent wellspring of a few minerals including magnesium. Every 100 grams (around 11 dried figs) offer 68 mg of magnesium. Figs likewise give manganese, calcium, potassium, and Vitamin K and B6!

QUINOA

Did you realize that quinoa is really a natural product, not a grain? It's actual! However, paying little mind to what you call it, quinoa is an incredible wellspring of magnesium with 64 mg for every 100 grams (that is a little over a large portion of a cup).

Quinoa used to simply be a vegetarian staple, however, now you can discover it on the menu of numerous standard cafés! A cup of cooked quinoa offers 8 grams of complete protein and every one of the nine fundamental amino acids — uncommon for non-creature protein. It additionally has 3.5 grams of sound fat and 5 grams of fiber.

EDAMAME

Like their highly contrasting bean family members, edamame (Also known as juvenile soybeans!) is a rich wellspring of supplements. Regarding magnesium, edamame presents 62 mg for every 100 grams, which approaches about a cup.

Edamame is a decent wellspring of vegetarian protein, solid fiber, cell reinforcements, and Vitamin K! In any case, its important there has been a great deal of debate encompassing soy lately and whether it's true sound for you

FISH

Some consider it the "chicken of the ocean" because of its white tone and gentle flavor. So fish is a decent choice for the individuals who are not colossal enthusiast of fish but rather still need to get their omega 3s

Fish is stuffed with magnesium with every 100 grams offering 64 mg of this fundamental mineral. Fish is additionally an incredible wellspring of Vitamin B12 — which you might be low on if you do not eat a lot of red meat!

TOFU

Tofu is the most notable wellspring of veggie lover protein. It's likewise an incredible method to load up on minerals including calcium, iron, manganese, selenium, copper, phosphorus and indeed, magnesium! For every 100 grams of tofu, you get around 60 mg of magnesium.

On top of being nutritious, tofu is exceptionally flexible. It assumes the kind of whatever you cook it in. So feel free to add some to a smoothie; marinade and throw in a Thai curry, or sear with a crunchy covering to make artificial chicken fingers!

AVOCADO

Avocados are acclaimed for being an incredible wellspring of sound monounsaturated fats, which can help lower cholesterol and improve heart health. Yet, they have numerous advantages past heart wellbeing as well.

Add a medium avocado to your plate of mixed greens or sandwich, and you'll devour 58.3 mg of magnesium!

This rich, smooth treat is additionally high in fiber, which represents 79% of the carbs in avocados. Simply a large portion of avocado has 4.5 grams of fiber, which can help control craving, feed well-disposed gut microscopic organisms, and lessen diabetes hazard. Also, avocados are high in protein and low in sugar. It's a Win, win situation!

OKRA

Have you attempted okra? This frequently disregarded veggie may help your heart and visual perception and decrease your danger of diabetes.

It likewise brags an extensive rundown Vitamins including A, C, K, and the majority of the B nutrients. It's thick in minerals like calcium, potassium, manganese, copper, and, obviously, magnesium. In particular, a 100 gram serving of okra gives 57 mg of magnesium.

So this nutritious veggie makes an incredible side dish and offers an increase in protein and fiber as well. Take a stab at throwing the units in oil and preparing and flame broiling them until marginally boiled!

WHOLE GRAIN CEREAL

You may realize that entire grain cereals are more grounded than handled cereals — for their protein-rich germ as well as for their higher mineral substance (magnesium included!).

Presently, supplement substance may fluctuate contingent upon which entire grain cereal you pick yet you can hope to get around 52.4 mg of magnesium per 1 cup. Likewise, this sort of oat can satisfy more than 20% of your everyday fiber needs!

PEANUTS

A few groups avoid peanuts due to sensitivity concerns. In any case, if it's protected to devour peanuts in your family, you ought to because they make them astonish wellbeing properties.

Broiled peanuts rival the cancer prevention agent substance of blackberries and pomegranate. They're more extravagant in cancer prevention agents than carrots and beets! One of these cell reinforcements is resveratrol — the celebrated polyphenol found in red wine — which offers numerous wellbeing defensive advantages.

Also, obviously, these scrumptious vegetables (indeed, they're viewed as a vegetable!) contain a lot of magnesium: 49.9 mg per one-ounce serving. They're likewise a magnificent wellspring of Vitamin B, copper, and heart-solid monounsaturated fats.

SCALLOPS

Scallops are a most loved shellfish in light of current circumstances — these delectable luxuries are over 80% protein! A 100-gram serving gives 24 grams of protein and only 137 calories. They're likewise a decent wellspring of magnesium (44 mg for every 100 grams) and potassium.

Scallops offer a liberal measure of selenium — a cell reinforcement mineral that both lethargic bone misfortune and supports bone-building. Indeed, a 100-gram serving has 25.5 mcg of selenium, which is more than 40% of your day-by-day necessity. Also, remember, they're an incredible wellspring of bone-solid omega 3 unsaturated fats as well.

PRUNES

Prunes have a ton to bring to the table in the wellbeing division. Since its dried-out natural product has gotten its water eliminated, the concentrated adaptation of energy and thick supplements contrasted with new organic product.

So although a few supplements like Vitamin C are lost during drying, magnesium content remaining parts high. Truth is told, every 100 grams of prunes (around 10 natural products) conveys 41 mg of magnesium.

Simply ensure you check the name for added sugar and additives when you're buying your prunes. You'll need to search for regular prunes with no sugar added. This natural product is truly fond of its own, and an excessive amount of sugar is not useful for your bones.

POTATO

Potatoes have gained notoriety for being undesirable. However, like with most food sources, if you eat them with some restraint and set them up yourself, there's no explanation they cannot be important for a sound eating routine.

Indeed, potatoes are a decent wellspring of fiber, potassium, Vitamin C, and Vitamin B6. Furthermore, obviously, they contain a sound measure of magnesium as well. In particular, one medium prepared potato offers 39 mg of magnesium.

So whenever you're longing for fries no compelling reason to keep down! Simply make them yourself so you can handle the salt substance, and heat them on the stove for a better form of this famous side dish.

BROWN COLORED AND WILD RICE

Whole grains are better than prepared grains as far as sustenance — and rice is no special case! In contrast to white rice, brown-colored and wild rice have their outside husks unblemished. Furthermore, these husks are stuffed with sound supplements. That is the reason earthy-colored and wild rice offers 37 mg of magnesium for every 100 grams.

To place that in context, that is not exactly a large portion of a cup of rice for a ton of magnesium. Truth be told, on the off chance that you cooked one cup of rice, you'd get 80.3 mg of magnesium! These sorts of rice are likewise plentiful in phosphorus, potassium, and multi-skilled Vitamin B.

SALMON

Salmon is all around adored for its unpretentious, invigorating taste. Also, as a little something extra, it's an exceptionally nutritious food! Past the extremely significant omega 3 unsaturated fats, salmon is thick in bone-sound minerals like potassium, selenium, and, obviously, magnesium.

For every 100 grams of salmon (not exactly a large portion of a filet), you get 37 mg of magnesium. Also, here's a pleasant certainty: Salmon's excellent pink shading comes from the carotenoids in their eating routine, similar to the cell reinforcement astaxanthin.

POLLOCK

Pollock is another famous fish choice. This gentle, white fish has a comparable flavor to haddock or cod and is now and again utilized in fried fish and French fries. Be that as it may, you'll need to heat yours in the stove or flame broils it in a prospect better dinner! Also, Pollock is for sure solid.

This fish is an extraordinary wellspring of lean protein, which as you may know is key for bone wellbeing. It's likewise low in immersed fat and high in great fats, omega 3s.

It's a rich wellspring of minerals including (you got it!) magnesium. For every 100 grams of Pollock, you get 37 mg of magnesium. So you'll certainly need to add this fish to the supper revolution.

SOY MILK

In case you're delicate to lactose or are simply hoping to eliminate dairy, soy milk is an incredible other option. It's liberated from soaked fat and wealthy in protein. Soy milk is generally strengthened with a portion of the very supplements that you get from customary milk like calcium, riboflavin, and Vitamin A and D.

However, soy milk should not be misleadingly sustained with magnesium since it's normally high in this bone-solid mineral! Indeed, some soy milk contains around 36.6 mg of magnesium.

Considering how it's made? It's basically water joined with ground soybeans (which clarifies its high magnesium content).

Simply check the name to ensure the soy milk you buy is produced using characteristic soybeans and not soy protein seclude (SPI) — a made variant of soy protein that does not give the entire food's advantages. Here's a brisk tip to help you differentiate: When soy milk is made normally, you'll generally discover the words "entire or whole soybeans" on the rundown of fixings.

LENTILS

Lentils are maybe most notable for their heart medical advantages. This supplement thick vegetable contains fiber, folic corrosive, and potassium — all of which support heart wellbeing. Lentils are additionally an incredible wellspring of protein, iron, and calcium, which clarifies why they're a staple for some vegans. Unexpectedly, these supplements are on the whole useful for your bones as well!

Furthermore, obviously, lentils are a decent wellspring of magnesium: 100 grams offers 36 mg. So why not join lentils into your supper plans? They make an extraordinary side dish, and nowadays, you can even discover solid, lentil-based pasta at the supermarket.

SHELLFISH

Shellfish are a sumptuous treat with some astonishing medical advantages. Like most fish, clams are high in aggravation battling omega 3 unsaturated fats. They're additionally plentiful in protein and bone-supporting minerals like calcium, iron, and selenium, zinc, and indeed, magnesium.

For every 100 grams (approx 10 eastern shellfish or three pacific clams), you get 36 mg of magnesium. Shellfish are an incredible wellspring of Vitamin B12 — a fundamental nutrient that supports nerve capacity and energy levels. Indeed, 100 grams of shellfish gives more than 6 times your everyday necessity of this nutrient!

ROCKFISH

Rockfish, additionally called Pacific red snapper and dark bass is a substantial white fish that is wealthy in omega 3s. A wide range of rockfish are a decent wellspring of magnesium and offer 33 mg for every 100 grams (somewhat less than a full filet).

Rockfish is likewise wealthy in bone-sound selenium — 100 grams would more than cover your day-by-day necessity of this mineral! At long last, this fish is an uncommon food wellspring of Vitamin D. Furthermore, obviously is urgent because it assists you with engrossing the calcium your bones need to remain solid, sound and crack-free.

KALE

Kale is another dull, verdant green that is gotten mains crack freely on account of its unbelievable wellbeing properties. Truth be told, numerous individuals consider kale a "super food". What's more, it's nothing unexpected when you consider this supplement force to be reckoned with contains more iron per ounce than meat!

It's additionally plentiful in numerous fundamental minerals for your bones, including calcium, potassium, and, obviously, magnesium. For every 100 grams of kale, you get 33 mg of magnesium. At last, it's significant that kale is high in nutrient K1 which is significant for making osteocalcin — a protein fundamental for bone wellbeing.

BULGUR

Bulgur is a lesser-realized entire grain produced using broke wheat. It's a more modest grain than rice — practically like a blend among couscous and quinoa. Furthermore, it's loaded with supplements that your body and your bones long for!

Regarding bone-sound minerals, bulgur is a decent wellspring of potassium, selenium, and indeed, magnesium. Every 100 grams of bulgur conveys 32 mg of magnesium. Bulgur is wealthy in fiber which upholds absorption and gut wellbeing.

BANANAS

Did you know the logical name for banana, Musa sapientum, which means "product of the wise man"? Furthermore, bananas are to be sure a shrewd natural product to remember for your eating regimen.

They're an incredible wellspring of bone-solid minerals including potassium and magnesium. Truth be told, they're perhaps the most extravagant wellspring of potassium in the world! Concerning magnesium, only one medium banana offers about 31.9 mg of this fundamental mineral.

YOGURT

Yogurt is a most loved breakfast, nibble, and even treats. So it's acceptable to realize it has some extraordinary medical advantages. It's wealthy in protein. It could be useful for assimilation. Furthermore, obviously, it contains numerous significant supplements... not least of which is magnesium!

In some entire milk yogurt, you get about 29.4 mg of magnesium. You likewise get a decent measure of calcium — around 296 mg for every cup.

Furthermore, you might need to reevaluate picking low-fat assortments of yogurt. The full-fat assortments offer more health benefits, and studies recommend they would not make you put on weight all things being considered.

Truth be told, a few long-haul contemplates have discovered that individuals who eat full-fat dairy will in general be less fatty and are more averse to get overweight.

Note that these investigations are co- relational, so they should be thought about while considering other factors! Be that as it may, they do uphold the incorporation of full-fat dairy in a solid eating routine.

HALIBUT

Halibut is a low-fat fish, so it does not have as many bone-solid omega 3 unsaturated fats as high-fat fish like salmon. Yet, it's as yet a brilliant wellspring of lean, top-notch protein, and it's abundant in nutrients and minerals.

A 100-gram parcel (not exactly a large portion of a filet) of halibut offers 28 mg of magnesium. It's likewise an extraordinary wellspring of nutrients including Vitamin D, A, and B nutrients like niacin (B3), pyridoxine (B6), and B12. These nutrients add to everything from mental capacity to calcium ingestion!

BROCCOLI

Numerous individuals consider broccoli one of the world's best food varieties, and the mark is merited!

Did you know the phytochemicals in broccoli are known for their disease defensive impacts? Broccoli is wealthy in bone-sound supplements like calcium, potassium, and magnesium. Truth be told, 100 grams (that is about a cup of crude broccoli), it conveys 21 mg of magnesium.

For those with joint torment, cruciferous veggies like broccoli are high in carotenoids (a type of Vitamin A). Carotenoids shield cells from fiery cytokines that separate collagen in joints and cause torment. What's more, the rundown of supplements goes on... broccoli is likewise a decent wellspring of fiber, the parent omega 3 unsaturated fat ALA, and Vitamin B, E, and A.

BRAZIL NUTS

Brazil nuts are one of a kind for likewise very high in selenium. Indeed, only two Brazil nuts give over 100% of the RDI for this mineral also; nuts are mitigating, advantageous for heart wellbeing, and can diminish hunger when eaten as tidbits

CHAPTER THREE

RESISTANT BOOSTING FOOD SOURCES AND NATURAL PRODUCTS

VITAMIN D RICH FOOD SOURCES

Vitamin D and Components for Decrease of microbial contamination, General digestion and Vitamin D exercises are additionally very much perceived. Inside the skin, Vitamin D3 is framed by the collaboration of UVB radiation moving toward 7-dehydrocholesterol all through the skin, joined by a warm response. The oral Vitamin D or Vitamin D3 is transformed into 25(OH) D in the liver and afterward into 1, 25(OH) 2D (calcitriol), hormonal metabolite in either the kidney or some other organ as wanted. The entirety of the effects of Vitamin D come from the passage of calcitriol into the atomic Vitamin D receptors, a DNA-binding protein that frequently discusses straightforwardly with controlling successions around explicit qualities and enlisted people dynamic chromatin edifices that hereditarily and epigenetically take part in transcriptional creation alterations. Some well-known job of calcitriol is simply to help deal with the serum calcium fixations, although it does in such a parathyroid chemical (PTH) criticism circle, which has numerous huge jobs in the living being itself. Different reports talk about how Vitamin D declines the danger of viral sicknesses. Vitamin D has a few pathways by which the threat of viral contamination and mortality is diminished. An investigation of the significance of Vitamin D in diminishing the basic virus hazard arranges these components in three classifications: versatile invulnerability, actual boundary and characteristic cell insusceptibility. Vitamin D assists with advancing hole intersections of tight, and intersections of followers (e.g., by E-cadherin). A few investigations tended to how infections harm the uprightness of the intersection, developing infection tainting just as other micro-organisms. Vitamin D improves cell natural resistance to some degree by inciting 1, 25-dihydroxy Vitamin D into antimicrobial peptides, similar to human cathelicidin, LL-37, and guards. Cathelicidins exhibits the solid antimicrobial action by an assortment of organisms including Gram-negative and Gram-positive microorganisms encased and un-enveloped infection and growth. Such host-derived compounds annihilate the unfamiliar microbes by obliterating their films and consequently can smother the endotoxin's organic exercises. As referenced in that, they have countless more capacities. In a mouse model, LL-37 diminished replication of flu kind of infection. A clinical report expressed that Vitamin D supplementation with 4,000 IU/d decreased disease with the dengue infection. Vitamin D likewise improves cell obstruction, by raising the cytokine storm that the intrinsic insusceptible framework causes. As found in COVID-19 patients, the natural safe framework creates both anti-inflammatory and pro-inflammatory cytokines in light of bacterial and viral irresistible infections. Vitamin D may diminish the improvement of pro-inflammatory Th1 cytokines, known as tumor corruption factor α and interferon ÿ. Vitamin D organization diminishes the creation of pro-inflammatory cytokines and improves the creation of anti-inflammatory cytokines by macrophages and their references. Vitamin D is a successful resistance modulator; 1, 25(OH) 2D3 invigorates reactions initiated by the T-helper sort of cell 1 (Th1), essentially by attempting to smother provocative cytokine creation IL-2 and interferon-gamma (INFπ). Additionally, 1,25(OH)2D3 energizes the advancement of cytokine by the T-helper type 2 (Th2) cells, which assists with improving the circuitous hindrance of Th1 cells by enhancing this with activities impacted by an assortment of cell types. Additionally, 1, 25(OH) 2D3 encourages actuation of T administrative cells and in this way restrains aggravation measures. Centralizations of serum 25(OH) D keep on declining with age that might be critical for COVID-19 as case casualty rates (CFRs) ascend with age; reasons incorporate lacking time spent in the daylight, and diminished nutrient D creation because of lower skin levels of 7-dehydrocholesterol. Moreover, certain professionally prescribed meds by invigorating the pregnane-X receptor decline serum 25(OH) D focuses are additionally managed. These incorporate anti-neoplastic, anti-epileptics, anti-inflammatory specialists, anti-toxins, anti-retroviral, anti-hypertensive, endocrine drugs, and certain natural prescriptions. The utilization of drugs tranquilizes ordinarily increases with age. Supplementation with Vitamin D additionally improves the creation of anti-oxidation-related qualities (glutathione reductase and subunit regulator glutamate-cysteine ligase). The expanded creation of glutathione saves the utilization of ascorbic corrosive (Vitamin C), which likewise has antimicrobial properties, and has been recommended for COVID-19 avoidance and treatment.

SOURCES OF VITAMIN D

THE VITAMIN D FROM SUNLIGHT

The premier snippet of data to value concerning Vitamin D is that it is known as 'The Vitamins from Sunlight '. This is because Sunlight is important for the blend of Vitamin D in the skin and those ailing in Sunlight are in high danger of inadequacy. We feel compelled to emphasize this point as much as possible as Vitamin D is not found in plenitude normally in food sources. So basically, insufficient sunlight resulting in insufficient Vitamin D, and henceforth issues with a far-reaching lack in certain pieces of the world (UK) especially in regions, for example, portions of Scotland that gets even less sunlight. The measure of sunlight (UV) in the cold weather months is deficient and they should draw on their real holds (accordingly).

There are a few food varieties abundant in Vitamin D and principally sleek fish and eggs anyway. Fish utilization is highest and has the Vitamin D Mission note:

Salmon and other slick fish are enormous in vitamin D, alongside liver, eggs, and sustained grains. But since of the amounts required it's difficult to get enough from diet alone."

VITAMIN D FOOD VARIETIES

Probably the most ideal approach to get sufficient nutrient D in your eating routine is to eat an assortment of good food varieties from the entirety of the nutritional categories, including some strengthened food sources. Likewise, focus on around 15 minutes of late morning sun openness, at any rate, two times seven days.

FOOD VARIETIES THAT GIVE VITAMIN D INCLUDE:

Global unit per serving

- Beef liver (cooked). 3 ounces: 42 IU.

•	Cereal, invigorated with 10% of the day-by-day estimation of nutrient D. 0.75 to 1 cup: 40 IU.

•	Cod liver oil. 1 tablespoon: 1360 IU.

•	Egg yolk. 1 enormous egg: 41 IU.

•	Margarine invigorated. 1 tablespoon: 60 IU.

•	Milk invigorated. 1 cup: 115-124 IU.

•	Orange juice invigorated. 1 cup: 137 IU.

•	Salmon (sockeye, cooked). 3 ounces: 447 IU.

•	Sardines (canned in oil, depleted). 2 sardines: 46 IU.

•	Swiss cheddar. 1 ounce: 6 IU.

•	Swordfish (cooked). 3 ounces: 566 IU.

•	Tuna (canned in water, depleted). 3 ounces: 154 IU.

•	Yogurt braced with 20% of the everyday estimation of nutrient D. 6 ounces: 80 IU.

FOOD SOURCES

Barely any food sources are normally abundant in vitamin D3. The best sources are the substance of greasy fish and fish liver oils. More modest sums are found in egg yolks, cheddar, and hamburger. Certain mushrooms contain some vitamin D2; plus, some industrially sold mushrooms containing higher measures of D2 due to purposefully being presented to high measures of bright light. Numerous food sources and enhancements are sustained with vitamin D like dairy items and oats.

- Cod liver oil

- Salmon

- Swordfish

- Tuna fish

- Orange juice sustained with vitamin D

- Dairy and plant milk braced with vitamin D

- Sardines

- Beef liver

- Egg yolk

- Fortified cereals

1. SALMON

Salmon is a famous greasy fish and an extraordinary wellspring of vitamin D.

As per the Nourishing specialists, Food Structure Data set, one 3.5-ounce (100-gram) serving of cultivated Atlantic salmon contains 526 IU of vitamin D or 66% of the DV.

Regardless of whether the salmon is wild or cultivated can have a major effect?

Overall, wild-gotten salmon packs 988 IU of vitamin D per 3.5-ounce (100-gram) serving or 124% of the DV. A few investigations have found much more elevated levels in wild salmon — up to 1,300 IU per serving (Nonetheless, cultivated salmon contains just 25% of that sum. All things being considered, one serving of cultivated salmon gives around 250 IU of vitamin D or 32% of the DV (

By and large, that is 124% and 32% of the DV, individually.

2. HERRING AND SARDINES

Herring is a fish eaten around the planet. It tends to be served crude, canned, smoked or salted.

This little fish is additionally perhaps the best wellspring of vitamin D.

New Atlantic herring gives 216 IU per 3.5-ounce (100-gram) serving, which is 27% of the DV (If fresh fish is not your thing, salted herring is additionally a decent wellspring of vitamin D, giving 112 IU per 3.5-ounce (100-gram) serving, or 14% of the DV.

Nonetheless, salted herring likewise contains a high measure of sodium, which a few groups devour a lot of.

Canned sardines are a decent wellspring of vitamin D too — one can (3.8 ounces) contains 177 IU, or 22% of the DV different kinds of greasy fish are additionally acceptable vitamin D sources. Halibut and mackerel give 384 IU and 360 IU per large portion of a filet, separately

3. COD LIVER OIL

Cod liver oil is a famous enhancement. On the off chance that you do not care for fish, taking cod liver oil can be crucial to getting certain supplements that are inaccessible in different sources.

It's an amazing wellspring of vitamin D — at around 448 IU per teaspoon (4.9 ml), it times in at a huge 56% of the DV. It has been utilized for a long time to forestall and treat inadequacy in kids Cod liver oil is in like manner an awesome wellspring of vitamin A, with 150% of the DV in only one teaspoon (4.9 ml). Be that as it may, nutrient A can be poisonous in high sums.

Consequently, be wary of cod liver oil, making a point to not take it excessively.

Additionally, cod liver oil is high in omega-3 unsaturated fats, which numerous individuals are lacking in.

4. CANNED FISH

Numerous individuals appreciate canned fish as a result of its flavor and simple stockpiling techniques.

It's likewise normally less expensive than purchasing fresh fish.

Canned light fish gets together to 268 IU of vitamin D in a 3.5-ounce (100-gram) serving, which is 34% of the DV.

It's likewise a decent wellspring of niacin and vitamin (Shockingly, canned fish contains methyl mercury, a poison found in numerous sorts of fish. On the off chance that it develops in your body, it can cause genuine medical conditions In any case, a few sorts of fish present less danger than others. For example, light fish is commonly a preferred decision over white fish — it's viewed as protected to eat up to 6 ounces (170 grams) each week.

5. EGG YOLKS

Individuals who do not eat fish should realize that fish is not the solitary wellsprings of vitamin D.

Entire eggs are another acceptable source, just as a magnificently nutritious food.

While the vast majority of the protein in an egg is found in the white, the fat, nutrients, and minerals are discovered generally in the yolk.

One common egg yolk contains 37 IU of vitamin D or 5% of the DV (Vitamin D levels in egg yolk rely upon sun openness and the vitamin D substance of a chicken feed. At the point when given a similar feed, field-raised chickens that meander outside in the daylight to produce eggs with levels 3–4 times higher.

Furthermore, eggs from chickens given vitamin D-enhanced feed may have up to 6,000 IU of vitamin D per yolk. That is incredible multiple times the DV Picking eggs either from chickens raised outside or showcased as high in vitamin D can be an extraordinary method to meet your everyday prerequisites.

Eggs from monetarily raised hens contain just around 37 IU of vitamin D per yolk. In any case, eggs from hens rose outside or took care of vitamin D-improved feed contain a lot more significant levels.

6. MUSHROOMS

Barring braced food varieties, mushrooms are the solitary acceptable plant wellspring of vitamin D.

Mushrooms can incorporate this nutrient when presented to UV light, Be that as it may; mushrooms produce vitamin D2, while creatures produce nutrient D3.

Despite the fact that vitamin D2 assists raising with blooding levels of vitamin D, it may not be pretty much as successful as vitamin D3

Regardless, wild mushrooms are superb wellsprings of vitamin D2. Truth be told, a few assortments get together to 2,300 IU per 3.5-ounce (100-gram) serving — almost multiple times the DV (30).

Then again, industrially developed mushrooms are frequently filled in obscurity and contain next to no D2.

In any case, certain brands are treated with bright (UV light). These mushrooms can give 130–450 IU of vitamin D2 per 3.5 ounces (100 grams).

Mushrooms can blend vitamin D2 when presented to UV light. Just wild mushrooms or mushrooms treated with UV light are acceptable wellsprings of vitamin D.

7. SUSTAINED FOOD VARIETIES

Common wellsprings of vitamin D are restricted, particularly in case you're vegan or do not care for fish.

Luckily, some food items that do not normally contain vitamin D are sustained with this supplement.

8. COW'S MILK

Cow's milk, the most ordinarily burned-through kind of milk, is normally a decent wellspring of numerous supplements, including calcium, phosphorous, and riboflavin

In few nations, cow's milk is invigorated with vitamin D. It ordinarily contains around 115–130 IU per cup (237 ml), or around 15–22% of the DV

9. SOY MILK

Since nutrient D is discovered only in animal product items, veggie lovers and vegetarians are at an especially high danger of not getting enough

Thus, plant-based milk substitutes like soy milk are frequently sustained with this supplement and different nutrients and minerals typically found in cow's milk.

10. SQUEEZED ORANGE

Consequently, a few nations invigorate squeezed orange with vitamin D and different supplements, like calcium

11. GRAIN AND CEREAL

Certain grains and moment cereal are likewise invigorated with nutrient D.

Despite the fact that sustained grains and oats give less vitamin D than numerous normal sources, they can, in any case, be a decent method to support your admission.

CHAPTER FOUR

IMMUNE BOOSTING FOOD VARIETIES AND ORGANIC PRODUCTS

VITAMIN C AND E RICH FOOD VARIETIES

Vitamin C is a significant part of improving immunity, for youngsters, grown-ups, or even old individuals. Organic products like oranges, papaya, kiwi, and guava are abundance in nutrient C and ought to be remembered for the eating routine. Additionally, a few vegetables like eggplant, chime peppers, beetroots, spinach, and cauliflower are known to be very rich in vitamin C and are useful for immunity. Green vegetables like broccoli, mushrooms, and even kale is a couple of immunity supporters that one can remember for his/her eating routine. They improve the immunity arrangement of more established individuals quickly. Berries can likewise be remembered for the eating regimen alongside food sources rich in omega-3 unsaturated fats—beans, flax seeds, and surprisingly a few nuts. Old individuals ought to devour Spirulina and Curcumin, as they are very abundance in vitamin C and minerals. These super foods help in building and fortifying immunity at an extraordinary level.

Water-soluble vitamins have critical advantages in the treatment of sepsis and septic stun, a life-threatening condition, which is brought about by irritation delivered by pathogenic living beings. Alternate ways vitamin C guides the body as a pro-oxidant for insusceptible cells, cancer prevention agent for lung epithelial cells, and immunosuppressive impacts. Food sources that contain vitamin C are oranges, kiwi, kale and broccoli.

Vitamin E is imperative for keeping up the general strength of older individuals, including their immunity. Vitamin E is an incredible cell reinforcement that can shield you from different contaminations, microorganisms, and infections. Drenched almonds, peanut butter, sunflower seeds, and even hazelnuts ought to be devoured to get the day-by-day portion of vitamin E. Vitamin E works basically as an un-specific, chain-breaking cell reinforcement that boycotts the spread of lipid peroxidation. This vitamin is frequently an extremist peroxyl scrounger that secures the polyunsaturated fats in plasma films and lipoproteins. F2-isoprostane evaluation is the best record of free-radical creation and oxidative lipid obliteration in vivo. The F2-isoprostane are improved, and their emanation might be decreased by taking enhancements with vitamin E. Vitamin E plays out a huge part in protecting insusceptible reactions, with a little insufficiency influencing resistance, or enhancements with rates higher than recommended, improving old individuals' humoral and cell-mediated immunity. These perceptions have built up an interest in whether vitamin E supplementation during substantial pressure can weaken immunosuppressant and oxidative pressure. Some work has shown that 1–5 months of supplementation with vitamin E (200–1200 IU dl – tocopherol) raises tocopherol plasma level yet has no negative effects athletic productivity of muscle harm lists brought about by compression and a differing impact on oxidative pressure brought about by work out. The dubious presence of these discoveries is connected to the investigation of plan issues, similar to the subjects' planning and sort of activity, readiness for age levels, the volume and state of the vitamin E supplement and strategies for oxidative pressure evaluation. The ROS–resistance relationship is as yet depicted; however developing proof shows a connection.

The age of ROS and the cancer prevention agent position were connected to immunity contrasts in some infection measures and the mending cycle, however, this cooperation is neglected in the human athletic exertion. In a prior examination by certain scientists, supplementation with vitamin C during an ultra-marathon did not impact oxidative pressure and invulnerable anomalies instigated by active work. In vivo vitamin C principally gives cancer prevention agent insurance as an extreme scrounger of peroxyl and oxygen in the fluid stage. We contended that although vitamin E restrains the spread of lipid peroxidation, the above multivitamin has a more prominent potential to go about as a cautious measure to changes in resistance and lipid peroxidation initiated by action than vitamin C.

The point was to survey the effect of vitamin E ingestion on oxidative pressure or invulnerable changes following the Marathon Big showdowns in Kona, Hawaii. Thirty-eight randomized, dual-blind marathon runners got vitamin E (800 IU dl D — tocopherol) just as fake treatment containers for a very long time until the occasion of the race. It is presumed that vitamin E enhancements would reduce physical activity-induced ascends in insusceptible adjustments in the feeling of serious inconvenience, oxidative pressure and fiery cytokines.

LEAFY FOODS THAT HAVE MORE VITAMIN C THAN ORANGE

There are a lot more food varieties that are higher in Vitamin C substance than even an entire orange, did you think about them? Peruse on to think about these food sources

Vitamin C substance is high in oranges, yet these different food sources and vegetables have the following features.

• Fruits and vegetables other than citrus organic products additionally have high Vitamin C

•	These are normally happening high source of Vitamin C

•	Fruits, for example, guava and vegetables, broccoli are a few sources

The significance of Vitamin C could not possibly be more significant, particularly so in the colder time of year. Aside from keeping up the generally speaking sound working of the body, this unassuming Vitamin has a few medical advantages. Orange and citrus natural products are evidently the rulers of Vitamin C as they are known to have the vitamin in high amounts. It is said that a solitary orange can satisfy a critical segment of your suggested dietary remittance of Vitamin C. Yet, did you realize that there are a lot more food varieties that are higher in Vitamin C substance than even an entire orange?

HERE ARE LEAFY FOODS THAT HAVE MORE NUTRIENT C THAN ORANGE:

1. GUAVA

Yellow and red natural products are typically credited with having high vitamin substance; however, guava is a natural product that stands tall as an exemption. A solitary guava natural product, gauging 100 grams, has over 200mg of Vitamin C substance (according to the USDA), which is twice pretty much as high as that in an orange.

2. PINEAPPLE

Pineapple is a misjudged supplement force to be reckoned with - the natural product contains gigantic measures of vitamin C. A mineral that is once in a while found in normal food varieties, manganese is additionally found in pineapple making it an incredible option to the eating routine.

3. STRAWBERRIES

Strawberries are known for their cancer prevention agent properties all finished; however, they are likewise a rich source of vitamin C. Their vitamin C substance is somewhat more than that in a solitary orange.

4. KIWI

In case you're searching for a solid nibble choice or an approach to add 'green' to your eating routine, Kiwi natural product is the best approach. Only one kiwi organic product contains up to 84mg of vitamin C, alongside other crucial nutrients like vitamin K and E.

5. MANGO

Mangoes are normally high in vitamin C and beta-carotene and consequently help in boosting immunity too. Green mangoes really have more vitamin C substances than their yellow or red partners.

6. PAPAYA

Papaya is best delighted in fresh, regardless of whether as a plate of mixed greens or as juice. A large portion of papaya, whenever eaten crude, gives an essentially higher measure of Vitamin C than a solitary orange.

7. BROCCOLI

Aside from being an incredible vegetable for keeping up in general wellbeing, broccoli is additionally an extraordinary normally happening source of vitamin C, which helps fix harmed tissue and keeping up sound immunity.

8. KALE

Kale has a few medical advantages, and one of them is in effect high in vitamin C and K. A delightful kale juice is the best approach to add to your eating routine or can even be supplanted in pesto sauce, instead of basil.

9. RED AND YELLOW RINGER PEPPERS

Red and yellow ringer peppers are super-wealthy in cell reinforcements, which help in keeping up eye and heart wellbeing. They likewise contain high measures of vitamin C, which supports collagen level and may assist with forestalling cellular breakdown in the lungs as well.

Thus, whenever you're searching for approaches to add to your eating regimen that are normally high in vitamin C, attempt one of these choices as opposed to utilizing the customary orange.

10. CANTALOUPE

Melon is a rich source of vitamin C, with 202.6 mg of the vitamin in a medium-sized melon and 25.3 mg in one cut.

11. RED CABBAGE

Red cabbage, additionally called purple cabbage, is high in vitamin C and low in calories. A half-cup contains just 14 calories yet practically 50% of the suggested every day estimation of vitamin C. It is likewise a rich source of fiber and different nutrients.

12. ORANGE

Some of the time called ascorbic corrosive; it upholds your insusceptible framework and helps your body utilize the iron its get from food. Your body additionally utilizes it to make collagen, a springy kind of connective tissue that makes up pieces of your body and recuperates wounds. What's more, it's a cancer preventive agent that shields your cells from harm. Men need 90 milligrams each day, and ladies need 75 milligrams. A medium orange has around 70 milligrams; however, numerous different food varieties are acceptable sources, as well.

13. TOMATOES

You'll get around 20 milligrams of vitamin C out of a medium tomato - on the off chance that you eat it raw. Vitamin C levels go down when you cook tomatoes. Yet, a cell reinforcement called lycopene goes up. So to get every one of the advantages, you may give new tomatoes a shot in your sandwich at lunch and prepared pureed tomatoes on your pasta for supper.

14. POTATO

A medium prepared potato has around 20 milligrams of vitamin C. What's more, they're useful for you. They're a superb source of potassium and fiber. Rather than boiling them in oil, attempt them stove simmered in olive oil. On a heated potato, trade the spread for better garnishes, as new salsa and low-fat cheddar.

15. CAULIFLOWER

A cup of florets has around 40 milligrams of vitamin C. It's additionally a respectable source of vitamin K, folate, and fiber. You can eat it raw, steam it, or dish it with a touch of olive oil. Spruce up the flavor with new spices, similar to thyme, which has around 4 milligrams of vitamin C in a tablespoon.

16. BRUSSELS FLEDGLINGS

They have 50 milligrams of vitamin C per 1/2 cup cooked, alongside a lot of vitamin K, fiber, and different supplements. Cook them with bacon and onions or only a tad of olive oil for a scrumptious, fulfilling side dish.

17. GRAPEFRUIT JUICE

A 6-ounce glass should give you 70 to 95 milligrams of vitamin C, about what you need for the afternoon. If you cannot stand the acrid taste, a similar measure of squeezed orange ought to do comparably well.

18. KAKADU PLUMS

The Kakadu plum (Terminalia ferdinandiana) is an Australian local super food containing multiple times more vitamin C than oranges.

It has the most elevated known grouping of vitamin C, containing up to 5,300 mg for every 100 grams. Only one plum packs 481 mg of vitamin C, which is 530% of the DV (3).

It's likewise rich in potassium, vitamin E, and the cancer prevention agent lutein, which may be of immense benefit to eye wellbeing. Kakadu plums contain up to 5,300 mg of vitamin C per 100 grams, making it the most extravagant known source of this vitamin. Only one plum conveys around 530% of the DV.

19. ACEROLA CHERRIES

Only one-half cup (49 grams) of red acerola cherries (Malpighia emarginata) conveys 822 mg of vitamin C or 913% of the DV

Humans contemplating utilizing acerola extricate have shown that it might have disease battling properties, help forestall UVB skin harm, and even diminishing DNA harm brought about by an awful eating regimen

Regardless of these promising outcomes, no human-put-together investigations concerning the impacts of acerola cherry utilization exist.

Only one-half cup of acerola cherries conveys 913% of the suggested DV for vitamin C. The organic product may even have disease battling properties, albeit human-based exploration which is inadequate.

20. ROSE HIPS

The rosehip is a little, sweet, tart natural product from the rose plant. It's stacked with vitamin C.

Around six rose hips give 119 mg of vitamin C or 132% of the DV (10).

Vitamin C is required for collagen blend, which supports skin respectability as you age.

Studies have discovered that vitamin C decreases sun harm to the skin, diminishing wrinkling, dryness, and staining and improving its general appearance. Vitamin C likewise helps wound recuperating and incendiary skin conditions like dermatitis. Rose hips give 426 mg of vitamin C per 100 grams. Around six bits of this organic product convey 132% of the DV and support better-looking skin.

21. BEAN STEW PEPPERS

One green bean stew pepper contains 109 mg of vitamin C or 121% of the DV. In correlation, one red stew pepper conveys 65 mg, or 72% of the DV (12, 13).

Also, stew peppers are wealthy in capsaicin, the compound that is answerable for their hot taste. Capsaicin may likewise decrease pain and aggravation, There is additional proof that around one tablespoon (10 grams) of red bean stew powder may help increase fat-consuming agents in the body. Green bean stew peppers contain 242 mg of vitamin C per 100 grams. Consequently, one green stew pepper conveys 121% of the DV, while one red stew pepper conveys 72%.

22. BLACKCURRANTS

One-half cup (56 grams) of blackcurrants (Ribes nigrum) contains 101 mg of vitamin C or 112% of the DV (20).

Cell reinforcement flavonoids known as anthocyanins give them their rich, dull tone.

Studies have shown that eating less of foods high in cell reinforcements like vitamin C and anthocyanins may decrease oxidative harm related to ongoing sicknesses, including coronary illness, malignancy, and neurodegenerative infections

Blackcurrants contain 181 mg of vitamin C per 100 grams. One-half cup of blackcurrants packs 112% of the DV for vitamin C and may help to decrease persistent aggravation.

23. THYME

Gram for gram, fresh thyme has multiple times more vitamin C than oranges and one of the greatest vitamin C centralizations of every culinary spice.

One ounce (28 grams) of new thyme gives 45 mg of vitamin C which is half of the DV (23).

Indeed, even sprinkling 1–2 tablespoons (3–6 grams) of new thyme over your supper adds 3.5–7 mg of vitamin C to your eating regimen, which can reinforce your insusceptibility and help battle contaminations?

While thyme is a famous solution for sore throats and respiratory conditions, it's likewise high in vitamin C which improves immunity wellbeing, make antibodies obliterate infections and microscopic organisms, and clear contaminated cells

Thyme contains more vitamin C than most culinary spices with 160 mg for every 100 grams. One ounce of new thyme gives half of the DV to vitamin C. Thyme and different food sources high in vitamin C lift your resistance.

24. PARSLEY

Two tablespoons (8 grams) of new parsley contain 10 mg of vitamin C, giving 11% of the suggested DV (26).

Alongside other verdant greens, parsley is a critical wellspring of plant-based, non-heme iron.

Vitamin C expands the assimilation of non-heme iron. This forestalls and treats iron-insufficiency sickliness. One two-month study gave individuals with vegetarian food regimen diet 500 mg of vitamin C two times every day with their suppers. Toward the finish of the examination, their iron levels had expanded by 17%, hemoglobin by 8%, and ferritin, which is then a put-away type of iron, by 12%

Parsley contains 133 mg of vitamin C per 100 grams. Sprinkling two tablespoons of new parsley on your supper conveys 11% of the DV for vitamin C, which assists increase with pressing ingestion.

25. MUSTARD SPINACH

One cup of crude hacked mustard spinach gives 195 mg of vitamin C or 217% of the DV (30).

Although the warmth from cooking brings down the vitamin C substance in food sources, one cup of cooked mustard greens actually gives 117 mg of vitamin C or 130% of the DV (31).

Likewise, with numerous dim, verdant greens, mustard spinach is additionally high in vitamin A, potassium, calcium, manganese, fiber, and folate.

Mustard spinach contains 130 mg of vitamin C per 100 grams. One cup of this verdant green gives 217% of the DV to vitamin C when crude, or 130% when cooked.

26. LEMONS

Lemons were given to mariners during the 1700s to forestall scurvy. One entire crude lemon, including its strip, gives 83 mg of vitamin C, or 92% of the DV (44).

The vitamin C in lemon squeeze likewise goes about as cell reinforcement.

At the point when products of the soil are cut, the compound polyphenol oxidase is presented to oxygen. This triggers oxidation and turns the food to earthy-colored. Applying lemon juice to the uncovered surfaces goes about as an obstruction, forestalling the searing cycle

Lemons contain 77 mg of vitamin C per 100 grams, with one medium lemon conveying 92% of the DV. Vitamin C has intense cell reinforcement benefits and can hold your cut leafy foods back from becoming earthy colored.

27. LYCHEES

One lychee gives almost 7 mg of vitamin C, or 7.5% of the DV, while a one-cup serving gives 151% (46).

Lychees additionally contain omega-3 and omega-6 unsaturated fats, which has immense advantage for your cerebrum, heart, and veins.

Studies explicitly on lychee are inaccessible. In any case, this organic product gives a lot of vitamin C, which is known for its part in collagen amalgamation and vein wellbeing

A Research investigation in 196,000 individuals tracked down that those with the most elevated vitamin C admissions had a 42% decreased danger of stroke. Every additional serving of organic products or vegetables brought down the danger by an extra 17%

Lychees contain 72 mg of vitamin C per 100 grams. One single lychee contains a normal of 7.5% of the DV for vitamin C, while a one-cup serving gives 151%.

28. AMERICAN PERSIMMONS

Persimmons are an orange-shaded natural product that takes after tomato. There is a wide range of assortments.

Although the Japanese persimmon is the most well-known, the local American persimmon (Diospyros virginiana) contains just about multiple times more vitamin C.

One American persimmon contains 16.5 mg of vitamin C or 18% of the DV (48).

American persimmons contain 66 mg of vitamin C per 100 grams. One American persimmon packs 18% of the DV for vitamin C.

FOOD SOURCES AND NATURAL PRODUCTS RICH IN VITAMIN E

1. SUNFLOWER SEEDS

Looking for a sound bite? All you need is a modest bunch of sunflower seeds to crunch on. Nutty, loaded with fundamental supplements including vitamin E, magnesium, copper, vitamin

B1, selenium, and a ton of fiber, will take you far. You can likewise embellish your typical chicken or fish serving of mixed greens with sunflower seeds, tidy up your eggs with this super seed or sprinkle a modest bunch on your one-pot dinners.

2. SPINACH

Viewed as one of the best green verdant vegetables, spinach is home to a few fundamental vitamins and minerals, particularly vitamin E. Simply a large portion of a cup of spinach has 16% of your day by day necessity of vitamin E. You can gobble spinach crude or prepare it up in servings of mixed greens.

Note to recall: Cooking spinach or steaming it before a supper can really expand the quantity of its supplements.

3. VEGETABLE OILS

Olive oil, sunflower oil, raw grain oil is among the best sources of Vitamin E. Did you know that only 1 tablespoon of raw grain oil holds 100% of your day by day admission of Vitamin E? What's more, 1 tbsp of canola oil contains 12% of the day by day vitamins esteeming needed by the body.

You ought to by and large evade vegetable oils, yet when you need to increase your vitamin E admission; these oils can be remembered for your usually solid eating routine.

4. PEANUTS

In the event that you love peanuts, you're in karma! Peanuts are an incredible source of cell reinforcements, wealthy in monounsaturated fats; help forestall colon malignant growth and gallstones, and useful for the heart as well. Truth be told, 1/fourth cup of peanuts contains 20% of the necessary vitamin E admission, and eating peanuts brings down the danger of weight acquire. As indicated by Nutritionist, Nut contains a specific cell reinforcement called resveratrol which has been known to battle free radicals that can cause coronary illness and malignant growth. So tidy up your commonplace Asian serving of mixed greens with peanuts or embellishment noodles and pan-sears with a modest bunch of peanut

5. AVOCADO

As per numerous source specialists, avocado is wealthy in fiber, low in carbs, stacked with carotenoids and only 1 avocado contains 20% of the necessary day by day admission of Vitamin E. Maybe probably the yummiest food with Vitamin E, avocados addresses nature's creamiest, oil-rich food. Remember avocados for your eating regimen by pounding it up as guacamole, adding not many cuts to your plate of mixed greens, or slathering it on toast with cherry tomatoes. You can launch your day to the sound path with heated egg and avocado.

6. ALMONDS

At the point when you need a convenient solution of energy, nothing beats a small bunch of almonds. 1 cup of almonds might be high in calories, however it gives double the important measure of Vitamin E for the day for example 181%. Not an aficionado of crude almonds? You can drink up a glass of almond milk or top off a toast

7. SHRIMP

We understand your opinion - fish is a source of cell reinforcements, indeed, shrimp might be high in cholesterol yet it is a low-calorie food that is rich in minerals and vitamins, particularly

Vitamin E. It is likewise high in vitamin D, vitamin B12, vitamin B3, selenium, and copper. How to appreciate shrimp to get the greatest vitamin E consumption? You can join shrimp with hacked onions, tomatoes, stew peppers, garlic, lemon juice, and a shower of olive oil on a bed of romaine lettuce.

8. HAZELNUTS

A brilliant source of vitamin E, hazelnuts contain 21% of the everyday suggested estimation of vitamin E each day, just as protein, vitamin A and vitamin C. Hazelnuts, are extraordinarily wealthy in folate and help lower LDL or awful cholesterol. They can be eaten all alone or added to treats, chocolates, cakes, and pies. You can likewise change it up a piece and appreciate hazelnut spread.

9. ASPARAGUS

Asparagus gives an interesting mix of calming properties just as vitamin C, beta carotene, zinc, manganese, and selenium. Indeed, 1 cup of asparagus contains 18% of your every day prerequisite of vitamin E. Asparagus likewise accompanies hostile to malignancy benefits, manages glucose and helps in processing. You can prepare an omelet loaded down with asparagus toward the beginning of the day or throw freshly cooked pasta with asparagus or simply sauté it with a solid blend of mushrooms, ringer peppers, and tofu with garlic.

10. BROCCOLI

This individual from the cabbage family is a decent source of protein and profoundly rich in vitamin E. Broccoli additionally contains hostility elements to disease properties, brings down awful cholesterol (LDL), and is outstanding amongst other detox food varieties. You can add some broccoli to soups or plates of mixed greens or serve steamed broccoli as a side dish during supper to make the most of its numerous medical advantages. To keep its wholesome properties unblemished, you should cook broccoli at a low cooking temperature.

11. PEANUT BUTTER (SMOOTH STYLE)

In spite of the fact that a little high in calories, peanut butter additionally contains fiber that guides weight reduction Peanut butter is likewise wealthy in magnesium that helps assemble bones. It additionally contains great fat.

You can apply peanut butter over whole grain bread and have it for breakfast. In any case, on the off chance that you are maintaining a strategic distance from grains or gluten, you can apply the nut spread to organic product or celery sticks. You can likewise take nut-based wafers.

12. PINE NUTS

The supplements in pine nuts additionally support energy. They are extraordinarily acceptable in magnesium too, the low levels which can prompt exhaustion.

You can utilize pine nuts in your pasta or as a sandwich spread. You can likewise add toasted pine nuts to plates of mixed greens for that additional crunch.

13. DRIED APRICOTS

Dried apricots contain moderate measures of eatable fiber just as a few fundamental vitamins, including vitamin E. The fiber in them helps in cholesterol guideline and absorption.

Furthermore, vitamin E upgrades hair and skin wellbeing. You can mix dried apricots in a natural product plate of mixed greens.

14. GRANOLA

Granola is a decent source of fiber just as a supplement that helps battle coronary illness, diabetes, and heftiness. It likewise contains omega-3 unsaturated fats (because of the nuts), which have a large group of different advantages – going from improved heart and mind wellbeing to better skin. You can have without grain granola for breakfast.

15. KIWIS

They are likewise rich in vitamin C that helps support immunity. They likewise contain serotonin, which helps treat sleep deprivation by prompting rest.

You can add kiwis to an organic product serving of mixed greens in the wake of blending in with yogurt.

17. TARO ROOT

Taro root is likewise wealthy in different cell reinforcements (beta-carotene and cryptoxanthin) that help vision wellbeing. The undeniable degree of vitamin C additionally helps support the resistant framework. You can substitute potato with taro root in your vegetable serving of mixed greens.

16. RED (OR GREEN) CHIME PEPPERS

Red ringer peppers additionally contain lutein and zeaxanthin, two cell reinforcements that add to eye wellbeing. They are additionally nice sources of iron and are rich in vitamin C (this supplement helps in iron ingestion), the two of which help forestall weakness. You can add finely hacked red chime peppers to your grain or verdant plates of mixed greens. You may even add them to your morning meal omelet.

18. PAPRIKA

Paprika is additionally wealthy in iron that assumes a part in energy age. What's more, the capsaicin in paprika is known to loosen up the veins and lower pulse. You can add a spoonful of paprika to your number one hummus for additional flavor. You can likewise prepare natively constructed soups with paprika.

19. TURNIP GREENS

While turnip greens taste somewhat harsh, they have an extraordinary portion of vitamin E and a few other essential supplements – one of them being vitamin C, which generally advances hair and skin wellbeing. Besides, it gives adequate folate also.

You can add raw turnip greens in sandwiches or plates of mixed greens. You can likewise take them bubbled or add them to your number one soups.

20. MUSTARD GREENS

Very much like Swiss chard, mustard greens are profoundly nutritious, giving numerous medical advantages. They are one of the top transporters of vitamin E, folate, and vitamin A, C, and K.

Despite the fact that they taste best when all around cooked, we suggest utilizing them in plates of mixed greens or considering standard cooking them to hold a large portion of their advantages.

21. MARGARINE

Margarine is rich in vitamin E as it is produced using vegetable oils. It likewise contains undeniable degrees of solid unsaturated fats and lower levels of immersed fats. These could be advantageous to your heart. In any case, certain brands of margarine may likewise contain Tran's fats, so check the names before you purchase. Additionally, go for those brands containing corn oil as it gives an additional portion of vitamin E.

You can supplant spread with margarine on your morning meal toast.

22. WHEAT (WHOLE GRAIN)

Whole grain wheat is likewise connected with sound weight reduction and a decreased danger of metabolic condition. It likewise is wealthy in magnesium, which assumes a significant part in diabetes treatment.

You can get ready entire grain plates of mixed greens (counting entire wheat) and have them for breakfast.

23. PAPAYA

Papaya likewise has incredible cell reinforcement properties that forestall various illnesses. It can even battle irritation and battle acid reflux.

You can add new papaya to your natural product smoothie for added fortification.

24. TOMATOES

Consider it an organic product or a vegetable, the tomato perpetually advances into our eating regimen in some structure. They are extraordinarily wealthy in lycopene, a cell reinforcement known to battle malignancy and various sicknesses.

You can add cut tomatoes to your sandwich, or even plan tomato soup for your evening supper.

25. GRASS-FED BUTTER

Grass-fed butter or margarine is one of only a handful few wellsprings of butyric corrosive, which is known to battle irritation. Notwithstanding vitamin E, the spread contains vitamin A – a supplement fundamental for your vision and skin. You can add grass-fed butter or margarine to your morning meal toast.

26. PARSLEY

Parsley helps battle other hazardous illnesses like disease and diabetes. It is likewise rich in vitamin K that adds to bone wellbeing. Although fresh parsley is better, you can likewise utilize dried ones promptly accessible on the lookout. You can basically toss a couple of twigs of parsley in your serving of mixed greens.

27. OLIVES

Use as an organic product or oil, olive is an extraordinary method of getting your day-by-day vitamin E portion. Olives likewise contain oleic corrosive that manages cholesterol levels and eventually improves heart wellbeing.

Add them to pizzas, servings of mixed greens, or pasta, or consider utilizing them alone with bread.

28. OREGANO

Oregano is known to show anti-cancer movement. It likewise contains intensifies that can help in diabetes therapy. You can utilize oregano as a plate of mixed greens besting or even join it in sandwiches. All things considered, that is with the rundown of vitamin E-rich food sources. There's uplifting news for individuals who favor meat. Chicken thigh is known to have the most elevated vitamin E content. This is trailed by chicken bosom and pork shoulder. The advantages of vitamin E (of the enhancements, particularly) can generally be seen uniquely in the individuals who endure an insufficiency.

29. SWISS CHARD

Swiss chard is a dim green verdant vegetable that contains 1.89 mg of vitamin E in a 100 g serving. In the same way as other verdant greens, Swiss chard contains a scope of extra supplements, including:

- 6116 IU nutrient A

- 81 mg magnesium

- 30 mg nutrient C

- 1.80 mg iron

- 379 mg potassium

- 1.6 g fiber

30. BUTTERNUT SQUASH

Butternut squash is a delectable vegetable regular in many fall and winter dishes. There is a 1.29 mg Confided in Wellspring of vitamin E in 100 g of prepared butternut squash.

31. BEET GREENS

While numerous individuals know about the flavor of beetroot, not every person realizes that it is feasible to eat the "greens" or leaves. Individuals can utilize beet greens in plates of mixed greens or sauté them in oil. A 100 g serving of cooked beet greens contains 1.81 mg Confided in Source of vitamin E.

Beet greens contain numerous extra supplements, including:

- 7654 IU nutrient A

- 24.9 mg nutrient C

CHAPTER FIVE

SPICES AND HERBS

A portion of the immunity-boosting spices is garlic, dark cumin, and licorice. Remember them for the eating regimen of the old as tea or by adding them to their food. This would not just upgrade their invulnerability however; it will improve their gut also. Homegrown treatment is very notable in Traditional or Customary Chinese Medication (TCM).

Conventional Chinese Medication has a long history and is a fundamental piece of the treatment or counteraction of certain episode sicknesses. The TCM intercession additionally accomplished a noteworthy helpful impact during the SARS plague in 2003. During the COVID-19 recuperation period, more than 3,100 TCM clinical staff was doled out to the region of Hubei just as the TCM program was remembered for the COVID-19 Testing and treatment Rule, and TCM experts were completely associated with the whole salvage measure. TCM's decoction,

Chinese brand name medication, needle therapy acupuncture, just as other trademark medicines were utilized widely and are fundamentally founded on the separation of the condition. Diverse TCM facilities were masterminded and the predetermined clinic was set up, while the TCM group is additionally altogether associated with the treatment. Presently, the complete number of genuine circumstances being taken care of by TCM has surpassed 60,107. In 102 instances of TCM signs that diminished clinical indication downfall time by 2 days, diminished internal heat level recuperation time by 1.7 days, diminished emergency clinic stays normal by 2.2 days, expanded CT picture improvement rate by 22%, expanded clinical endurance rate by 33%, the clinic stay rate diminished by 27.4 percent just as 70% increase in lymphocyte. Furthermore, in the treatment of genuine TCM patients, the real length of administration in the medical clinic, just as the hour of a nucleic corrosive transmission hurtful, was abbreviated by over 2 days.

Traditional or Customary Chinese Medication zeroing in on a general significant reason for COVID-19 pneumonia patients, may have helpful solutions, similar to those of gancaoganjiang decoction, qingfeipaidu decoction (QPD), qingfeitouxiefuzhengrecette, sheganmahuang decoction, and so on qingfeipaidu decoction which included, Polyporus Gypsum Fibrosum, Armeniacae Semen Amarum Cinnamomi Ramulus, Atractylodis Macrocephalae Rhizoma, Poria, Alismatis Rhizoma, Glycyrrhizae Radix et Rhizoma Praeprata cum Melle, Scutellariae Radix, Bupleuri Radix, Zingiberis Rhizoma Recens, Asteris Radix et Rhizoma, Pinelliae Rhizoma Praepratum cum Zingibere et Alumine Farfarae Flos, Rhizoma, Aurantii Fructus Immaturus, Belamcandae, Asari Radix et Rhizoma, Dioscoreae Rhizoma, Pogostemonis Herba, and Citri Reticulatae Pericarpium the COVID-19 demonstrative and treatment plan has been presented as the overall remedy in China. Of the 701 announced cases took care of with QPD, 130 cases were effectively treated and delivered from the clinic, 51 clinical manifestations blurred, 268 instances of afflictions assisted with improving, and 212 instances of non-aggravated stable indications. QPD's valuable endurance rate against COVID-19 surpasses 90%. COVID-19's objective area truly is the lung as indicated by the TCM hypothesis and the pathology trademark is "muggy and poison plague." The pharmacology examination of the organization showed that QPD has a total regulatory effect over multi-target and multi-component. Maybe, the essential pharmacological site is the lung, since 16 lung meridian spices show that decoction is principally explicit to lung sickness. This can likewise perform Dehumidification jobs rise and fall through spleen and stomach, just as show kidney, heart, and different organs assurance. One of the forthcoming indicated screens; large numbers of non-expressed with ACE-2, the COVID-19 particle can restrain COVID-19 replication by following up on various ribosomal proteins.

COVID-19 can add to setting off the resistant framework just as an ostensible expansion in irritation. Investigation of practical enhancement has shown that QPD can hinder and alleviate ill-advised invulnerable framework reaction and eliminate the disease by attempting to control the pathway related to cytokine activity and the immune-related pathway. Also, by anticipating patchouli liquor, atomic docking, shionone, and ergosterol, were found to have a decent anti-COVID-19 impact in the equation, which gives new substance mixtures to the improvement of new medications.

Here, to demonstrate its adequacy, we take for instance one distinguished COVID-19 patient took care of with TCM. Not many days before the start of the disease, the male patient was likewise on a working visit in Wuhan. Fever and hack have been continued during the confirmation stretch of time and respiratory rales were additionally not apparent for the two lungs. Western anti-infection agents were first utilized, for example, taking ganciclovir intravenous implantation, oseltamivir phosphate case orally, and recombinant inward breath of human interferon a1b vaporized. Although the nucleic basic analysis became negative, the consequences of chest CT uncovered that there was an expanded combination of two lung glass obscurity and expanded thickness, which was considerably more mind-boggling than induction. Serious sickness is related to the presentation of the patient's moist-heat condition just as the temperature is substantially more extreme than moistness; QPD has been applied for finding.

Conventional Chinese Medication has its own credits, similar to separation treatment, Yin and Yang balance, jumble separation, all-encompassing idea, reinforcing body protection from microbial factor end. TCM should have many years of involvement with body checking and pandemic opposition, with new points of view and involvement with treatment and counteraction. TCM's initial mediation can keep the sickness from changing over into serious and vital diseases for gentle and common patients. In genuine cases, by improving diseases, TCM has acquired the chance to safeguard them. COVID-19 restoration practice has shown that previous time TCM activity is a basic method of improving fix rate, shortening illness course, postponing infection movement, and limiting passing rates. Furthermore, the motivation behind why TCM works was not exclusively to forestall the contamination, yet additionally could forestall the infection, direct the invulnerable framework, advance body fix, and cutoff the incendiary tempest.

What's more, COVID-19's avoidance and control gauges completely mirror the preventive treatment of sickness belief system. Notwithstanding the pandemic illnesses recorded during the Han Administration, TCM's preventive measures ought to likewise incorporate games, brain rescarch, medicine, and diet.

In COVID-19's treatment and counteraction, this should offer the advantages of TCM in separating disorder and lessens both medical conditions and death rate. Moreover, logical exploration on the TCM with clear recuperating adequacy of COVID-19 should likewise be dropped to completely assess its instrument of activity and profound comprehension of COVID-19.

KITCHEN SPICES AND HERBS WITH A SAFE BOOSTING PUNCH

1. GARLIC

Garlic gives gentle antiviral, antibacterial, and disinfectant properties and is depicted as 'natures own anti-infection'. Taking garlic supplements over winter was appeared in one examination to decrease the odds of getting a bug by 63% and to accelerate recuperation in the individuals who were infected. In another investigation, matured garlic extricate was appeared to animate the expansion of two sorts of safe cells (regular executioner cells and Immune system microorganisms), bringing about diminished seriousness of colds and influenza). Smashing garlic and eating it raw or softly cooked will hold its intensity.

Garlic's forces work out in a good way past making food taste flavorful. Its idea to invigorate the insusceptible framework and lift the viability of white platelets, however, examines is uncertain.

Garlic is truly simple to utilize — eat it consistently to keep you feeling first class. Up your garlic admission when you're really wiped out, as well. Make a very garlicky soup (don't hold back on the bone stock, either), two or three raw garlic cloves, cook a garlic bulb, or pack it into a container of nectar and let it sit for half a month to implant.

Dietary portions of garlic are really protected. It is hard to take enough to hurt you, yet in case you're on the enemy of thickening meds, be mindful. (Also, brush your teeth if you wind up going extravagantly with raw garlic, as well!)

2.. GINGER

Ginger invigorates course, which thusly improves infection opposition. Because of its warming and antimicrobial properties, it's a fantastic spice for warding off ailments.

Mesh fresh new ginger into cereal or yogurt, toss some into your smoothie, or blend it into a warming tea.

3.   TURMERIC

Turmeric is antimicrobial, calming, and a cancer prevention agent — all significant lifts to the invulnerable framework.

It's typically a vital fixing in curries, effectively added to rice and quinoa dishes or stews, scrumptious in drinks like lassi or aged tonic, and I for one love sprinkling turmeric on my popcorn.

4.   CINNAMON, CLOVES, OREGANO, ROSEMARY, AND THYME

These promptly accessible kitchen spices and flavors all go about as cancer prevention agents, with mitigating, anti-infection, and hostile to contagious properties!

Add some zest to your colder time of year cooking and lift your immunity framework simultaneously.

IMMUNE BOOSTING HERBS AND SPICES FOR TEAS, COLORS, AND ENHANCEMENTS

1.   GREEN TEA

Green tea has numerous advantages however is generally known for its cell reinforcements, polyphenols, and flavonoids — all substances that help the insusceptible framework and help secure against colds and influenza.

Promptly accessible all over the place, this is a simple one to add to your everyday system. You could even blend it in with a couple of different spices to make your own resistant boosting tea mix!

2.   RED CLOVER

This modest weed is really an incredible medication. It is loaded with nutrients, loosens up pressure and stress, and battles colds and influenza.

It develops for all intents and purposes all over the place, and blooms are effortlessly gathered, dried, and put away for tea.

3. GINSENG

American ginseng is a striking spice with numerous utilizations, including assisting the body with recuperating physical and enthusiastic pressure. This makes it an incredible resistant framework supporter.

It is additionally known for its energy-boosting properties, ideal for the instance of the colder time of year blahs.

4. ASTRAGALUS

This realized immunity supporter helps the body ward off sickness. In addition to the fact that it increases resistance, yet it assists with revamping and reestablishing the insusceptible framework after ailment.

It is generally promptly accessible either in a container, tea, or color structure.

Utilizing promptly accessible spices to support your invulnerable framework can help you get wintertime ailments far from yourself and your family.

5. ELDERBERRY

Odds are, you've effectively attempted elderberry in some structure or another, as this profound purple berry has certainly gone standard in the previous few years.

Likewise called Sambucus, elderberry is antifungal, antibacterial, and antimicrobial, so it's acceptable at taking out any sort of muck you have going on. There's proof that elderberry is viable at treating seasonal influenza, also.

Its most normally found as a syrup (it will make your kitchen smell divine on the off chance that you Do-It-Yourself), yet colors (a plant separate made with liquor or glycerin), tablets, and even chewy candies can work as well.

Medical experts advised taking this cure once each day if you're attempting to forestall ailment, and considerably more much of the time once you're as of now wiped out — like clockwork or something like that.

Elderberry is viewed as protected, yet does not chug an entire container or anything like that — a teaspoon to a tablespoon of syrup at once. Keep syrups in the cooler, as they are not racking stable. If you have any immune system problems, it's most likely best to remain away (because it invigorates the resistant framework).

6. ECHINACEA

Another notable insusceptible promoter is echinacea, also known as coneflower. It works by animating the resistant framework to deliver characteristic executioner cells and other infection contenders.

A 2015 meta-investigation inferred that echinacea may be of immense benefit to people with low safe capacity the most, in any event, lessening the danger for a virus up to 35 percent.

Medical expert also recommends echinacea is most successfully utilized right when you begin to feel that tickle at the rear of your throat, as opposed to when an out and out affliction has grabbed hold.

Color is the most ideal approach to take it however teas would not bomb you either (particularly since you'll be hydrating your framework meanwhile). Search for Echinacea angustifolia or an entire plant extricate, because it's the most artificially bio-available (handily consumed and utilized by the body).

It's critical to take note of that on the off chance that you have ragweed hypersensitivity, you may likewise be touchy to echinacea — so on the off chance that you feel any obvious sensitivity indications like irritation, hives, or expanded clog, quit taking it right away.

On the off chance that you have an immune system issue, skip echinacea.

7. FIRE JUICE

This extraordinary fluid, here and there likewise called the Expert Tonic, is kitchen medication at its best: a serious combination of garlic, ginger, onion, horseradish, and hot peppers (in addition to quite a few other invulnerable boosting fixings like turmeric, or scrumptious ones like lemon or rosemary) marinated in apple juice vinegar.

Fire juice gets its adequacy from the shared force of this sinus-clearing, warming, disease bottling plant — in addition to an additional lift from the matured ACV. Also, indeed, this resistant mix will consume (positively!) going down.

It's ludicrously simple to make, so prepare a group and prepare it on your plate of mixed greens each night, sprinkle it on rice or quinoa, or make an effort when you feel a virus going ahead. On the off chance that handcrafting is not your jam, you ought to have the option to discover some from a nearby botanist or at a characteristic food store.

Stay away from this herb if you have GERD or a past filled with stomach ulcers.

8. ADAPTOGENS

You've likely heard this wellbeing world trendy expression over the most recent couple of years — adaptogens — however, may not be sure about what precisely it implies.

Basically, adaptogens are remedial spices that help the body in fighting and adjusting to pressure. They're incredible to use for individuals who become ill frequently or in the midst of hefty pressure, travel, or additional openness to microbes (as opposed to for regular upkeep or avoidance).

Ashwagandha, reishi (the two of which animate your infection battling lymphocytes, or white platelets,) and heavenly basil (invigorates the safe framework and battles infections) are generally acceptable decisions for invulnerable help

Purchase reishi as a powder and blend it into anything you're eating or drinking — it's protected to take in little portions (like a scoop of powder or a spurt of color). Same for ashwagandha — although avoid ashwagandha in case you're taking thyroid chemicals like Synthroid.

Heavenly basil can be made into a mixture and improved with nectar, It is prudent not to be taken if and when you're pregnant, however, Discover some different alternatives and attempt a couple and see which ones work for you.

At the point when the world is managing the lethal Covid-19, it is important to play it safe to keep yourself shielded from getting infected. This is the reason you need a solid insusceptible framework. Solid immunity assumes an imperative part in keeping the illness-causing infection and microbes from you and lessens the danger of falling debilitated. Individuals with bargained resistance regularly become ill and surprisingly their indications are more extreme when contrasted with others. There are various approaches to improve your resistance framework, preparing your body to battle any unfamiliar microorganisms. You can do it by making some way of life changes or by including some invulnerability boosting food things in your eating regimen

9. GILOY

Giloy is a flexible spice used to make Ayurvedic medications for quite a while. It assists with eliminating poisons from the body, decontaminates the blood, and battles sickness-causing microbes. Giloy contains oxidant properties that improve wellbeing help boost immunity and assimilation. Blend 15-30 ml of Giloy juice in a glass of water and devour it on an unfilled stomach in the first part of the day.

10. CHIA SEEDS

The little chia seeds are wealthy in cell reinforcements and omega-3 unsaturated fats, which are advantageous for upgrading insusceptibility. It likewise diminishes irritation and manages incendiary reactions in the body.

You can make chia seeds pudding to build your admission.

11. PUMPKIN SEEDS

Stacked with zinc, iron, and nutrient E, pumpkin seeds are useful for boosting safe capacity. Pumpkin seeds likewise are hostile to parasitic and against viral properties. It helps in cell development, improves your temperament and is surprisingly better for quality rest. Sprinkle some pumpkin seeds on your serving of mixed greens to receive its astounding wellbeing rewards.

12. SUNFLOWER SEEDS

Sunflower seeds are a rich source of vitamin E and supplements. The little crunchy seeds contain selenium which helps the body battle specific kinds of disease and assists with building your resistance. The cell reinforcement and vitamin E in the sunflower seeds battle free revolutionaries and are even useful for your skin. Add it to your serving of mixed greens or cereal.

13.. REISHI

Reishi, otherwise called Lingzhi, is a sort of mushroom. Reishi mushrooms contain beta-glucans, which are accepted to animate various sorts of cells in the invulnerable framework, including monocytes, common executioner cells, and dendritic cells. By invigorating these cells, they are better ready to distinguish and fend off diseases.

There's even some proof that the beta-glucans in reishi have powerful effects against tumor impacts, halting the development of disease cells, notwithstanding, more exploration should really comprehend the advantages of resihi mushrooms.

You can purchase reishi powder or cases to devour.

14. GOLDENSEAL

Goldenseal (Hydrastis Canadensis) is a lasting plant local to eastern North America.

Its foundations and leaves have been utilized in customary medication to treat an assortment of illnesses, particularly those including diseases or aggravation.

Today goldenseal positions among the most mainstream natural cures around the world. Teas, homegrown concentrates, or cases sourced from this plant are utilized to treat colds, roughage fever, stomach-related issues, sore gums, and skin issues Goldenseal is likewise added to different over-the-counter cures, for example, ear drops, ladylike cleanliness items, eyewash plans, cold and influenza cures, sensitivity alleviation items, purgatives, and stomach-related guides .

The spice is normally wealthy in a class of alkaloid compounds, with berberine, hydrastine, and canadine being found in the most noteworthy fixations.

These alkaloids are connected to antibacterial and calming properties and are accepted to be the fundamental purpose for goldenseal's implied medical advantages.

ADVANTAGES AND BENEFITS

Goldenseal is commended for its antibacterial and calming properties. It's regularly taken to forestall or treat upper respiratory parcel infections and the normal cold

It's likewise used to treat skin issues, absence of craving, hefty or difficult periods, sinus infections, acid reflux, and other incendiary or stomach-related issues In any case, research supporting its advantages is restricted and for the most part feeble.

15. ALOE VERA

Who knew an aloe vera plant had such a lot of goodness stuffed into its leaves? Despite the pack of supplements inside the gel, current science has looked to affirm numerous cases made about the plant. Specialists say the gel is not endorsed for any oral uses fundamentally because of an absence of proof. Analysts have gone through many years investigating the plant as a wellbeing cure and have thought of captivating outcomes.

Aloe's capacity to detoxify helps hold the resistant framework under control. The body has a greatly improved possibility at fending off disease and contamination if whatever number of supplements would be prudent can advance into the circulatory system.

Polysaccharides are the essential part of aloe vera gel. These mixtures, which are found in plants, make the thick nature of the gel.

A portion of these plants intensifies feed the insusceptible framework.

These equivalent fixings in aloe can likewise bother the safe framework, however not in an unsafe way, all things being equal, and the insusceptible framework increase since it considers these to be a danger. Nonetheless, polysaccharides are positively not a poison.

It's the normal motivation behind why individuals who eat plants have a decent resistant framework.

Moreover, the cell reinforcements that are available in the gel avoid free revolutionaries which contrarily sway resistance.

16. HONEY OR NECTAR

•	Excellent to build strength and perseverance.

•	Used by competitors as a perseverance food with stunning outcomes.

•	Extremely wholesome – it has every one of the amino acids the body needs.

•	Helps oxygen arrives at the synapses, reinforces hair like dividers.

•	Build protection from infections

•	Good for skin effectively affects the blood

•	Regulates intestinal capacity.

•	Helps the immunity framework, ordinary hair development can be diminished by insufficiency of amino acids from nectar.

THE PRIMARY BENEFITS OF HERBS AND SPICES

i. STIMULATES THE BODY INVULNERABLE FRAMEWORK---
Spices help to advance the body's normally happening useful material.

ii CLEANSING IMPACTS

It purifies and decontaminates the body without results

iii. EXTREMELY HEALTHFUL

Spices are high in nutrients, minerals, and different supplements and fabricate the body.

ii.

iii. NORMALIZES BODY CAPACITY

Spices control and tone the organs to work regularly.

v. RAISES ENERGY LEVEL OF THE BODY

Permit the body to have additional energy to keep up great wellbeing.

CHAPTER SIX

LIFESTYLE AND WAY OF LIFE

1. EAT A SOUND EATING REGIMEN

The supplements you get from food—specifically, plant-based food sources like natural products, vegetables, spices, and flavors — are fundamental for keeping your invulnerable framework working appropriately. Many plant-based food sources additionally have antiviral and antimicrobial properties, which help us, fend off disease.

For instance, research shows that flavors like clove, oregano, thyme, cinnamon, and cumin contain antiviral and antimicrobial properties that forestall the development of food-ruining microbes like Bacillus subtilis and Pseudomonas fluorescens, destructive growths like Aspergillus flavus, and anti-microbial safe microorganisms like Staphylococcus aureus, Besides, the zinc, folate, iron, selenium, copper, and vitamin A, C, E, B6, and B12 you get from the food you eat are the supplements your immunity framework needs to execute its work. Everyone assumes an interesting part in supporting resistant capacity.

Examination proposes, for instance, that inadequacy may improve the probability of infection, Our bodies do not create this fundamental, water-solvent vitamin all alone, so we need to get it through food sources, (for example, citrus organic products, kiwis, and a few cruciferous vegetables). You can get 95 milligrams (mg), or 106% of the day-by-day vitamin C you need by eating on a half-cup of red pepper.

Protein is likewise basic for safe wellbeing. The amino acids in protein help assemble and keep up resistant cells and holding back on this macronutrient may bring down your body's capacity to battle diseases. In one investigation by researchers, mice that ate an eating regimen comprising of just 2% protein were more seriously affected by this season's virus than mice that ate an "ordinary protein" diet with 18% protein. Yet, when analysts began taking care of the principal bunches an "ordinary protein" diet, the mice had the option to dispose of the infection.

With regards to an eating regimen that upholds great immunity wellbeing, centers around consolidating more plants and plant-based food sources. Add foods grown from the ground to soups and stews, smoothies, and servings of mixed greens, or eat them as bites. Carrots, broccoli, spinach, red ringer peppers, apricots, citrus natural products (like oranges, grapefruit, tangerines), and strawberries are on the whole incredible sources of vitamin A and C, while seeds and nuts will give protein, vitamin E, and zinc.

Extra sources of protein and zinc incorporate fish, lean meat and poultry according to the Institute of Sustenance and Dietetic

2. MONITOR PRESSURE

As per clinical specialists, long-haul pressure prompts persistently raised levels of the steroid chemical cortisol. The body depends on chemicals like cortisol during transient episodes of stress (when your body goes into a "battle or flight" reaction); cortisol has a valuable impact of really keeping the insusceptible framework from reacting before the upsetting occasion is finished (so your body can respond to the quick stressor).

In any case, when cortisol levels are continually high, it basically hinders the resistant framework from getting going and managing its responsibility to shield the body against expected dangers from germs like infections and microorganisms.

There are numerous powerful pressure decrease methods; the key is to discover what works for you. The proposal of contemplation (applications like Headspace and Quiet can help), journaling, and any action that you appreciate (like fishing, playing golf, or drawing). Attempt to do in any event one pressure diminishing action each day. In a rush start little. Put to the side five minutes sooner or later every day for entertainment only and increase it when you can.

3. GET A LOT OF GOOD QUALITY REST

Your body mends and recovers while you rest, making sufficient rest basic for a solid safe reaction.

All the more explicitly, rest is the point at which your body delivers and circulates key safe cells like cytokines (a sort of protein that can either battle or advance irritation), Lymphocytes (a kind of white platelet that manages safe reaction), and interleukin 12 (a favorable to incendiary cytokine).

At the point when you do not get sufficient rest, your resistant framework may not do these things too, making it less ready to shield your body against hurtful trespassers and making you bound to become ill. One investigation found that contrasted and sound youthful grown-ups who did not have rest issues, in any case, solid youthful grown-ups with sleep deprivation were more helpless to this season's virus even after getting immunized.

Lack of sleep additionally hoists cortisol levels, which obviously is likewise not useful for safe capacity. Our resistant framework wears out accordingly and we will, in general, have [fewer] stores to fend off or recuperate from disease."

Clinical specialists have exhorted that all grown-ups ought to get at any rate seven hours of rest each night to enhance wellbeing. To guarantee you get quality rest, focus on great rest cleanliness: Mood killer the gadgets, at any rate, a few hours before bed, and evade brutal or distressing books or discussions.

4. EXERCISE ROUTINELY (OUTSIDE, WHENEVER THE SITUATION ALLOWS)

Ordinary exercise brings down your danger of creating persistent sicknesses (like corpulence, type 2 diabetes, and coronary illness), just as viral and bacterial diseases, Exercise likewise builds the arrival of endorphins (a gathering of chemicals that diminish torment and make sensations of delight) making it an extraordinary method to oversee pressure. "Since stress adversely impacts our safe framework, this is another way exercise can improve safe reaction.

And keeping in mind that there is some proof that exceptionally long or extreme exercise meetings may stifle the resistance framework, making you more vulnerable to ailment and disease in the hours following your exercise, the proof on that question is opposing, as per similar Outskirts in Immunology audit. What's more, the epidemiological proof is abundant (contemplates that followed human conduct and results) showing that more dynamic individuals in general will have lower rates of both intense sicknesses (like diseases) and ongoing ones (like malignancy and type II diabetes). Studies that have seen what exercise means for the body on a cellular level propose that episodes of active work may make your insusceptible framework more cautious by dispersing safe cells all through your body to search for harmed or tainted cells.

Grown-ups ought to get at any rate 150 minutes (over two hours) of moderate-power vigorous exercise (like strolling, running, or cycling) or 75 minutes (one hour and 15 minutes) of focused energy oxygen consuming activity (like running) each week. You ought to likewise be doing strength preparing in any event double seven days.

Note: Greater action is connected to considerably more medical advantages, so reach skyward.

For considerably more invulnerable framework benefits, Clinical specialists suggest taking your activity outside. Investing energy in nature has appeared to help temperament, lower pulse, decrease aggravation, and backing invulnerable framework wellbeing, agreeing

Daylight additionally helps vitamin D in the body, which assumes a critical part in resistant wellbeing, as well.

5. WITH REGARDS TO LIQUOR, PRACTICE CONTROL

Drinking high measures of liquor is related to a scope of negative wellbeing impacts, including brought down immunity capacity. At the point when you drink high measures of liquor, your body is excessively bustling attempting to detoxify your framework to waste time with typical invulnerable framework work.

Significant degrees of liquor utilization can debilitate your body's capacity to battle disease and hinder your recuperation time. Therefore, individuals who drink high measures of liquor face a more prominent probability of pneumonia, intense respiratory trouble condition, alcoholic liver infection, and certain malignant growths, as indicated by a similar survey.

On the off chance that you do not as of now drink, do not begin. On the off chance that you drink once in a while, limit your liquor utilization to one beverage (comparable to a 4-ounce glass of wine) each day in case you're a lady and two beverages in case you're a man

6. TRY NOT TO SMOKE CIGARETTES

Like liquor, cigarette smoking can likewise influence resistant wellbeing. Anything that is a poison can bargain your insusceptible framework.

Specifically, the synthetics delivered by tobacco smoke — carbon monoxide, nicotine, nitrogen oxides, and cadmium — can meddle with the development and capacity of insusceptible cells, similar to cytokines, Lymphocytes, and B cells, Smoking likewise demolishes viral and bacterial contaminations (particularly those of the lungs, similar to pneumonia, influenza, and tuberculosis), post-careful diseases, and rheumatoid joint inflammation (an immune system sickness wherein the resistant framework assaults the joints.

Try not to smoke. Furthermore, keep away from used or secondary smoke at whatever point conceivable.

On the off chance that you presently smoke, there are numerous assets accessible to help you reduce your propensity to smoke, including advising, nicotine substitution items, solution non-nicotine prescriptions, and conduct treatment.

7. MONITOR INDICATIONS OF CONSTANT CONDITIONS

Ongoing conditions like asthma, coronary illness, and diabetes can influence the invulnerable framework and increase the danger of contaminations.

For instance, when individuals with type 2 diabetes do not deal with their glucose appropriately, this can make a constant, second-rate incendiary reaction that debilitates the body's safeguard framework.

Likewise, individuals with asthma are more helpless to getting — and surprisingly passing on from — influenza, and frequently experience more terrible influenza and asthma indications because of the disease, living with an ongoing condition can resemble attempting to drive a vehicle that has just three tires, On the off chance that you become ill with an infection, it will require more exertion for your body to recuperate.

If you deal with your ongoing conditions better, you'll let loose more holds to help your body fend off infection. So make certain to keep steady over any meds, specialist visits, and solid propensities that keep your manifestations under control. Your insusceptible framework will much be obliged.

150

CHAPTER SEVEN

CELL REINFORCEMENTS OR ANTIOXIDANTS

*T*his has been treated in early parts however it was not treated profoundly so allowed us to save a section for it, for information purpose.

Glutathione is an incredible cell reinforcement in the body, it searches for harming free radicals and is associated with tissue fix, and constructs synthetic compounds and proteins that are utilized for the invulnerable framework. N-Acetylcysteine, or NAC, advances the creation of glutathione and is likewise utilized as an enhancement. Studies in animals' models of other viral infections have shown that NAC decreased the seriousness and length of side effects by expanding cell guard and fix. NAC is taken in dosages of 500-600 mg. Glutathione can be taken orally 500 mg or by IV 400–2400 mg with a physician's instruction.

Quercetin is a bioflavonoid found in an assortment of foods grown from the ground. Animal and research facility examines have exhibited that quercetin can hinder a wide scope of infectious diseases including a COVID-19-related virus, SARS CoV. Quercetin upholds cell reinforcement limits and ensures lung tissue. As an enhancement is joined with vitamins C, bromelain is sold as a solitary enhancement. The suggestion is somewhere in the range of 500 and 1000 mg day by day. Significant sources are verdant green vegetables, dill, peppers, apples, grapes, fennel leaf, red onion, oregano, bean stew pepper, green tea, and dark tea.

Cancer prevention agent Rich in Food sources to lift Your Invulnerable Framework

Aggravation is a significant invulnerable framework. In any case, when wild, it can cause genuine harm. Irritation has been connected to significant illnesses like Alzheimer's, joint pain, malignant growth, diabetes, coronary illness, and indications of maturing.

There is s uplifting news, however: numerous food varieties are normally calming. Cancer prevention agents found in food varieties shield your cells from the impacts of free radicals and can help decrease an excess of irritation in your body.

Ocean growth, which has calming properties, contains multiple times more calcium by weight than milk.

HERE ARE CHARACTERISTIC, CALMING FOOD VARIETIES:

1.   BEETS

With their great red tone, they are amazing cancer prevention agent

 Beets can support your energy and lower your circulatory strain. A solitary serving of 500 milliliters of beetroot juice has been appeared to diminish pulse by 10.4/8 millimeters. Beets are high in nitrates; this investigation showed that a serving of beetroot juice supported athletic execution by one to three percent.

2.   BLUEBERRIES

These have been found to lessen irritation in numerous examinations on animals; there are yet to be more investigations done on people. Studies do demonstrate that blueberries are useful for cerebrum wellbeing. It is ideal to eat natural berries since pesticides on berries are difficult to wash away because of their size.

3.   BROCCOLI

It is stacked with detoxifying cancer prevention agents. Broccoli is especially rich sources of kaempferol and isothiocyanates, both calming phytonutrients. Discovery has shown the capacity of kaempferol to diminish the effect of hypersensitivity-related substances on our bodies. Broccoli even has a lot of omega 3 unsaturated fats, which is notable as a calming agent.

4. FLAXSEED

Oil has equilibrium of omega 3 and 6 unsaturated fats. The omega 3 unsaturated fats decrease aggravation. Exploration examines show lignans can moderate the development of prostate malignancy cells. It was likewise discovered that lignans may assume a significant part in expanding bosom disease endurance. Three examinations following many ladies determined to have bosom disease affirmed this.

4.   GREEN TEA

It contains numerous mitigating flavonoids. A recent report tracked down the most bountiful catechin of green tea (epigallocatechin-3-gallate) to be an intense calming compound with helpful potential. The cell reinforcement properties of green tea are successful to the point that reviews have shown a 22 percent diminished danger of creating bosom malignancy, a 48 percent decreased danger of prostate disease, and an astonishing 57 percent decreased danger of colorectal disease.

5.   GARLIC

It can help diminish aggravation. An investigation completed by researchers in North America uncovered that they discovered garlic to be multiple times more powerful than two anti-toxins at battling the Campylobacter bacterium—one of the reasons for intestinal sickness.

6.   GINGER:

Ginger decreases irritation and controls glucose. Ginger tea is an extraordinary expansion to any eating routine. An investigation distributed by clinical specialists contrasted ginger concentrate with normal torment executioners and discovered ginger to be powerful in lessening torment.

7. EXTRA VIRGIN OLIVE OIL

It helps battle irritation. Olive oil is loaded with polyphenols which shield the heart and veins from aggravation.

8. ONIONS

It contains quercetin, a powerful cell reinforcement that can help your body battle irritation. Onions invigorate the respiratory lot and help remove sputum (mucus). The onion is likewise demonstrated cell reinforcement and may help treat certain tumors.

9. SEAWEED

It contains a mind-boggling starch called fucoidan that reviews have appeared to decrease aggravation. Kelp contains multiple times more calcium by weight than milk. Kelp, kombu, wakame, and arame are acceptable wellsprings of ocean growth.

11. SPINACH

This is one of the greatest supplement thick food varieties. It contains an exceptional combination of phytonutrients, is high in cancer prevention agents and mitigating parts which help secure against cell harm.

12. TURMERIC

It has mitigating properties and is more compelling than calming drugs. Curcumin, the dynamic fixing in turmeric, focuses on numerous means in the fiery pathway at the atomic level.

EXAMPLES OF CELL REINFORCEMENTS AND ANTIOXIDANT THAT COME FROM OUTSIDE THE BODY INCLUDE:

- Vitamin A

- Vitamin C

- Vitamin E

- Beta-carotene

- lycopene

- lutein

- Selenium

- Manganese

- zeaxanthin

Flavonoids, flavones, catechins, polyphones, and phytoestrogens are a wide range of cell reinforcements and phytonutrients, and they are totally found in plant-based food varieties.

Every cancer prevention agent serves an alternate capacity and is not tradable with another. This is the reason it is essential to have a fluctuated diet.

FOOD SOURCES

Pomegranate is one source of cancer prevention agents.

The best sources of cell reinforcements are plant-based food sources, particularly products of the soil.

Food varieties that are especially high in cancer prevention agents are frequently alluded to as a "super food" or "useful food."

To acquire some particular cancer prevention agents, attempt to remember the accompanying for your eating regimen:

Vitamin A: Dairy produce, eggs, and liver

Vitamin C: Most foods grown from the ground, particularly berries, oranges, and chime peppers

Vitamin E: Nuts and seeds, sunflower and other vegetable oils, and green, verdant vegetables

Beta-carotene: Splendidly shaded leafy foods, like carrots, peas, spinach, and mangoes

Lycopene: Pink and red foods grown from the ground, including tomatoes and watermelon

Lutein: Green, verdant vegetables, corn, papaya, and oranges

Selenium: Rice, corn, wheat, and other entire grains, just as nuts, eggs, cheddar, and vegetables

DIFFERENT FOOD VARIETIES THAT ARE ACCEPTED TO BE ACCEPTABLE SOURCES OF CANCER PREVENTION AGENTS INCLUDE:

- Eggplants

- Legumes, for example, dark beans or kidney beans

- Green and dark teas

- Red grapes

- Dark chocolate

- Pomegranates

- Goji berries

Goji berries and numerous other food items that contain cancer prevention agents are accessible to buy on the web.

Food sources with rich, dynamic tones regularly contain the most cancer prevention, agents.

The accompanying food sources are acceptable sources of cancer prevention agents

- Blueberries

- Apples

- Broccoli

- Spinach

- Lentils

CHAPTER EIGHT

CONCLUSIONS AND FUTURE POINT OF VIEW

Individuals with low insusceptibility are more inclined to this world pandemic named COVID-19. To help or lift immunity, plant-based food sources assume a fundamental part by advancing advantageous microorganisms in the body. Different vitamins like C, D, and E are explored to give significant viewpoints to improving resistance. Natural products like oranges, papaya, kiwi, and guava are plentiful in vitamin C, while vegetables like eggplant, chime peppers, beetroots, spinach, and cauliflower are known to be very rich in vitamin C and are useful for resistance. An essential micronutrient is utilized in DNA union and cell multiplication, which control inborn and versatile safe reactions.

Vitamin D improves cell opposition, mostly by raising the cytokine storm that the natural resistant framework causes. Green vegetables like broccoli, mushrooms, and even kale are a couple of resistance sponsors that improve the invulnerable arrangement of more seasoned individuals quickly. Additionally, some spice mix in TCM is likewise known to assume a pivotal part in the counteraction of COVID-19. Future parts of this record for more examination which is required altogether on actual practices or practices and their job in immunity-related gives consequently forestalling COVID-19 perspectives. More exploration is needed to discover about the conduct of Covid-19 and the part of food in its counteraction. Immunity-boosting food mixes ought to be considered which, in the mix, given one and one makes health care-givers jobs. In nutshell, green food varieties are crucial against novel Covid-19 by improving the immunity of every matured gathering.

www.ingramcontent.com/pod-product-compliance
Lightning Source LLC
Chambersburg PA
CBHW060053260726
48658CB00004B/1280